Winning the Losing Battle
A True Story of Weight Loss and Transformation

Erica L. Bartlett

Winning the Losing Battle

A True Story of Weight Loss and Transformation

Erica L. Bartlett

Catching Words Press
Portland, Maine

Catching Words Press
Portland, Maine
www.rediscoveringfoodmaine.com
erica.l.bartlett@gmail.com
Copyright © 2015 Erica L. Bartlett

ISBN: 978-0-9862953-0-0

Photos are from the author's personal collection.

Book and cover design: Kitty Werner, RSBPress, Waitsfield, Vermont

Disclaimer: This is my story as I remember it. The names of a few individuals have been changed to protect their privacy. Some of the journal entries have been tweaked for clarity but are otherwise unedited from their initial writing.

Publisher's Cataloging-In-Publication Data
(Prepared by The Donohue Group, Inc.)

    Bartlett, Erica L.
     Winning the losing battle : a true story of weight loss and transformation / Erica L. Bartlett.

     pages : illustrations ; cm

    Issued also as an ebook.
    ISBN: 978-0-9862953-0-0

    1. Bartlett, Erica L.--Health. 2. Overweight persons--Biography. 3. Obesity--Psychological aspects. 4. Weight loss--Psychological aspects. 5. Food habits--Psychological aspects. 6. Autobiography. I. Title.

RC628 .B37 2015

362.1963/98092 B

This book is dedicated to my parents.

To the memory of my mother, Polly Bartlett,

wishing she could be here to see it.

And to my father, Erik Bartlett,

in thanks for all the support

and the chocolate chip cookie recipe.

Prologue

I pause, trying to catch my breath as I lean against a boulder. Then I make the mistake of looking ahead and groan. The steepest part of the Abol Trail remains before us, a field of rocks left by glaciers. It reminds me of how much further we have to go, when weariness, heat, and thirst already threaten to overwhelm me.

Climbing Katahdin is hard.

Then, as if it weren't anything at all, my brother Jeremiah blows past me, green cap almost jaunty on his head, his round, freckled face intent. Mom follows, her long, dark braid swinging over one shoulder. She gives me a quick, encouraging smile in passing, her eyes an enigma behind polarized lenses. Only Dad remains behind, capturing the day on his new toy, a camcorder.

I stare up at Mom, who has turned to wait for me. "How can you get up there?" Even the short question leaves me breathless, and my own long braid feels unusually hot and heavy on my back.

"Well, my legs are a little longer than yours." Mom puts it politely. Her third-grade students almost match her five feet, but at age ten, I stand a few inches shorter still. Jeremiah, at twelve, has surpassed both of us, and Dad has the greatest advantage at a whopping 5' 5". But I have quickly learned that when hiking, every inch counts.

"And you remember all those walks I took up and down the Hacker's Hill? There's a reason I did that." Mom's laugh sounds self-deprecating as she reminds us what she put herself through.

I sigh. I'd spent the summer doing my usual swimming and dog-walking, but nothing more intensive. If I had known when I agreed to the hike what this would truly be like, I might have done more. Or I might have opted out altogether. Why did I think I could climb a mile-high mountain, going over many miles of mostly steep, rocky terrain?

We continue climbing, but my energy lags. "It's just a little further," Mom says countless times. It doesn't take long for me to stop believing her. "Why don't you have a few peanut M&M's?" is another favorite phrase. That one I don't mind, as I never tire of candy.

But the sugar only does so much to combat the sheer effort of lifting my feet and legs again and again. Once I achieve the tree line, I don't even have the benefit of shade, just my visor keeping my own freckled face out of the sun. I want to give up. How had Jeremiah done this the year before? I knew they went up a different trail, but still, he made it to the top.

Now I knew why he said he'd admire me if I climbed Abol. At the beginning it had been great motivation, since I have spent much of my life trying to live up to his example. Now I don't even care.

Eventually Dad takes more drastic measures. Stopping and looking directly at me, bearded face stern and glasses also dark, he says, "Now, I'm not saying this to be mean, but we simply can't keep stopping to rest every few feet. I've said it before, but we really need to pick up the pace. It's a matter of time."

I don't have to respond because Mom says, "Erik, I've told you and *told you* to go on ahead."

"Polly, I'm talking to Erica."

"I know, but we've already been through this."

I squirm as their discussion continues, hating to cause dissent. I want to be able to charge ahead, but I know I don't have it in me to give the concerted effort Dad wants. It would almost be easier to go back.

Except—I can see the top of the rockslide, and I know the plateau waits just after, with Thoreau Springs offering a chance to refill my water bottle. Level ground! Fresh water! It sounds too good to be true. Swallowing, I tell myself I can go that far, despite the sun and my queasy stomach and my jeans that don't want to stretch as much as they need to.

I also don't want to admit my size might be holding me back. My chubbiness, cherubic in infancy and cute in young childhood, now proves a liability. A doctor had recently even told us that, at my height and age, 104 pounds was a cause for concern, something I refused to believe. Besides, Jeremiah is a bit heavy, too, and Dad's belly has recently started growing. If they can do it, so can I.

It helps when Dad and Jeremiah *finally* charge ahead. Mom and I press on but stop often. She starts carrying my backpack in addition to her own. For a little while, I move faster. But at the next stop, I am almost ready to cry.

"My water's gone."

Mom checks her own bottle. "You can have a little of mine, but we need to keep some until we get to the springs."

Before I can panic, a tall, rangy, bearded hiker approaches on his way down. He looks at me kindly. "Did I hear you say you don't have any water?" I nod shyly. "I refilled at the spring and have plenty. If you give me your bottle, I can fill you up."

"Thank you." I take a small sip when I get it back. It tastes amazing.

"Yes, thank you so much. Are you sure you'll be okay?" Mom asks him.

He smiles. "I'll be fine. After all, it's all downhill from here."

My spirits lift. We continue on, and I discover I like scrambling over some of the rocks, using both hands and feet for traction. One boulder in particular proves fun, falling as it had across two other rocks, with just enough space for me to crawl underneath. I emerge from the other side, both Mom and I laughing.

At last we reach the plateau. I expect the last mile to Baxter Peak to be simple, a level stroll after all the uphill. But the cold air at 5,000 feet knifes through my wet T-shirt, making me shiver. Even when I put my mittens and sweatshirt back on I can't stop shaking. The smaller rocks also make footing somewhat treacherous, requiring constant attention.

My brief burst of energy fades away. I continue, carried forward only by Mom's will and inertia. I barely even register when we join Dad and Jeremiah at the top. I simply find shelter from the wind in some rocks and collapse, wanting to be left alone with my grapes and more peanut M&M's.

My parents have other ideas.

Dad comes over with the camcorder running, while Mom crouches next to me with her 35mm camera. "How are you doing?" she asks.

"It was too hard." The words, quiet and on the verge of tears, slip out before I realize it. I didn't mean to confess that. I quickly eat another M&M.

"But you liked parts of it." I nod reluctantly as she reminds me of the good moments. "And I'm very proud of you. I know it's hard, but I'm glad you made it."

I nod again, this time feeling a little better. When she takes a picture, I even try to put some emotion into my expression, though after all the years of being photographed by Dad I have my automatic smile down pat.

She lowers the camera. "In a few minutes, I want to get a picture by the sign, okay?"

"Okay."

Then, mercifully, they leave me alone. I steadily munch on grapes and trail mix, this time more than just the peanut M&M's. Slowly my energy returns, and with it a dawning realization. I have actually reached the summit!

I emerge from my hidey-hole and join Jeremiah on a nearby rock. He smiles at me, braces glinting in the sun. "You made it. I thought you probably would."

I smile back, pleased. At least he hadn't doubted me, or not much. "Yep."

"Look at the way you can see the shadows of the clouds moving over the ground. I've never seen anything like it."

For the first time I perk up and take in the stunning view. The sky gleams a brilliant deep blue, while the sun beams on the jewel-like ponds and lakes glittering below. The lower forests look almost velvety green, and the rocks present a subtle yet lovely palette of earth tones, brown and gray and umber. An eagle circles below us, and the clouds themselves look close enough to touch.

My heart quickens with excitement. I've done it! I climbed Katahdin!

This time I don't mind posing for pictures. We stand by the sign marking the summit, the northern end of the Appalachian Trail. Then I start back down cheerfully. When we get to some of the huge boulders that caused me so much trouble before, I quickly slide down them, excited at the speed and ease of descent, landing with a "ta-da!" and little bow.

The agony of the way up recedes. By the time we have dinner, with delicious, homemade blueberry pie for dessert, I know I will do better on the hike next year.

Never once do I think I won't climb to the top of Katahdin again until I am twenty-seven, or imagine the tragedy and struggle it will take for me to complete that journey.

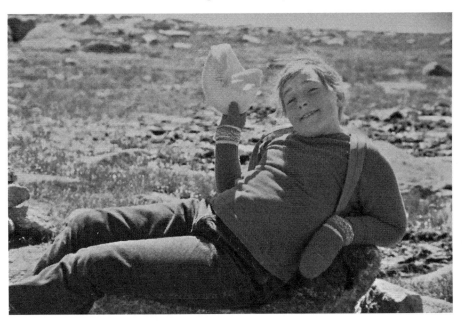

1986, Erica at the top of Katahdin

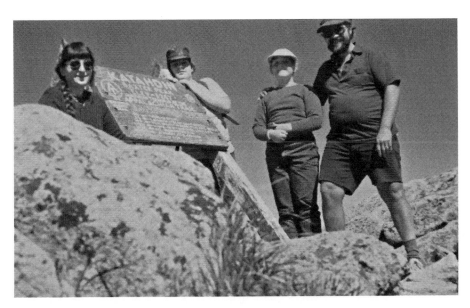

1986, L-R: Polly, Jeremiah, Erica, and Erik at Baxter Peak

Part 1 Tipping the Scales

1 Shapedown

January 1992 — age 15, 200 pounds

March 20, 1991

As I write this I am quite tired, and, frankly, quite sick of being overweight. I have lost twenty pounds since last summer, but really need to lose forty or fifty more.

It's just so hard! I try to tell myself that the momentary gratification I get from eating is not worth this continual feeling of despondency and disgust that inevitably comes. Yet, almost all my life I have eaten what and when I wanted, not caring about my weight, and that makes it very difficult to change my habits. Also, there are almost always sweets around, since Dad is much like I and enjoys baking. The other problem is that he is a very good baker; everything he makes is delicious.

"Erica, are you almost ready? We need to leave in about ten minutes."

I started as Mom's voice came from the other side of my bedroom door, interrupting my reading of old journal entries.

"Yeah, I'll be right there."

I sighed as I said it, reluctant to leverage myself up from where I had been lying on my bed, on my stomach. I'd meant to do some writing, working on fantasy stories, but instead found myself revisiting reflections about my weight.

With those thoughts in mind, the painful irony of reading my March entry at that moment did not escape me. Here I planned to embark on yet another weight-loss venture, and what did Dad do? Make brownies. Even at the opposite end of the house from the kitchen, the smell of fresh, warm chocolate wafted down to me. Still, it didn't surprise me. He only gave up baking those few times when he attempted to lose weight himself. Not that my life became any easier during those times, as another entry reminded me.

15

October 18, 1991

I've gone back and read previous entries, and suddenly realized how fickle I was. Numerous times, I've said that I was going to definitely lose weight, yet have I? No! And to tell the truth, I'm getting a little disgusted with myself. So this time, it's for real. I keep thinking of how fat I am, and if I actually look at myself, I'm sickened. So I'll avoid certain foods and start to work out again. Maybe I'll even lose weight.

At least, I hope. Of course, part of it is that Dad's losing weight, and I'm terrified to think that a time might come when I'll weigh more than anyone else in the house. I weigh 172-174 at present, and by the end of the year want to get back down to at least 164. Of course, I'd be overjoyed if I was around 159, but I don't know that it'll happen. I will try, though, and keep myself informed through this book.

Also, if I go to church youth conferences again, which I most definitely will, I want to be thinner to make a better impression. Yes, I'm starting to care what certain people think about me, and I do want it to be a high opinion. That's easier if you're thin.

My heaviness settled over me like an extra gravitational field. I hadn't lost weight since October. In fact, I had gained. How did it get this bad? But I knew the answer, if I chose to be honest with myself. The latest twenty pounds, for instance, I could clearly trace.

It started after a chiropractor adjustment in November, when Dr. Lindsey said, "Erica, I've noticed you've gained some weight."

I didn't like the sound of this. Up until then, she had avoided any real discussion of my weight, allowing me to feel safe and comfortable with her. Now, wary, I sat up quickly from tying my sneakers. She didn't need to see how the bulk of my stomach and breasts obscured my view when I bent over, or how even that modest effort quickened my breathing.

"I'm concerned about the effect on your back and hips, especially with your scoliosis, so I wanted to offer some suggestions about things you could do to lose weight."

She proceeded to rattle off ideas: eat less meat, more fish, fewer processed foods, more fruits and vegetables. I sat and listened, growing steadily more furious, feeling humiliated and betrayed. Nothing she said came as a revelation. I knew full well what I should be doing. Having her spell it out made me feel like a child. More, it raised my hackles to have anyone tell me what to eat.

So what did I do? The exact opposite. I sighed again. Yep, brilliant me, rebelling against advice I interpreted as judgment. Twenty pounds appeared almost magically.

I knew this, so why had I agreed when Mom asked if I wanted to try the Shapedown program? When I went into the kitchen to put on my boots and coat, though, I remembered.

"I think you'll like Betty." Mom practically beamed as she flipped her long hair out of her coat and put on her hat. Even bundled up, she didn't come close to my bulk.

"I hope so."

At the very least, if I went and made even a modest attempt to follow the program, it meant maybe Mom would stop getting on my case about my weight. That had to be worth something.

We arrived at the office in Portland, where a woman—slender, of course— greeted us. Not that I expected anything different from a nutritionist. At least she didn't have a model-thin body, all angles and sharp bones, only a normally slim one like Mom's.

Her fashionable clothes, though, made me conscious of my own attire. My long tunic over a turtleneck, falling shorter in the front because of my large chest, untucked to avoid drawing attention to my lack of a waist. My homemade skirt, which at least had the virtue of falling evenly because my aunt Patrice and I cut it longer in the back, providing enough material to cover my ample backside. My leggings under the skirt, not very old but already wearing thin on the inner thighs where my legs constantly rubbed together. I couldn't even imagine wearing pressed slacks and a button-down, tucked-in top with patterns.

I came out of those thoughts when she offered her hand with a smile. "You must be Erica. My name is Betty. It's a pleasure to meet you."

The smile looked genuinely friendly. "Nice to meet you, too." I shook her hand quickly, on alert for the recoil I usually expected from anyone touching me. After all, I knew how monstrous I had become. How could I not, when I so often saw the disgust reflected in others' eyes when they looked at me?

She didn't seem to notice, simply motioned me to the chair opposite the one she took. "Please, have a seat."

As I sat, I couldn't help comparing this to the visits with the counselor Mom made me see a couple years before. Betty's office was bright and homey rather than dim and cavernous, and she didn't sit across the room from me like she wanted to avoid me. I liked this better.

"Your mom has probably told you something about Shapedown, but I'd like to explain a little more. The goal of these meetings isn't to tell you what you should eat or how much. I'm here to help you think about why you eat when you do, how you feel about eating and exercise, and how I can help you learn new habits. How does that sound?"

"Good." In fact, it almost seemed too good to be true.

"I'd like to start by having you close your eyes. Imagine what it would be like to lose weight. What would you look like? How would you feel physically?"

Despite all my earlier attempts, I'd never done this. I closed my eyes and pictured myself getting smaller, lighter, my body becoming more like Mom's. It almost seemed as if I might float away.

When I told Betty, she said, "That's a great image because you know it's achievable and realistic, not trying to be like an actress or model. You can open your eyes, and now, if you don't mind, I'd like to have you tell me about why you think you gained weight, why you might eat too much, and if you have any goals for weight-loss."

The last part seemed simplest, the first idea coming to mind easily after my earlier thoughts on wardrobe. "Well, for goals I'd like to be able to buy clothes more easily, and ones that actually fit, and feel comfortable wearing a bathing suit. But what I'd *really* like to do is to be able to climb Mt. Katahdin again."

"Why is that?"

I sought for the words to describe my complex mix of emotions. "My family goes camping at Baxter State Park every summer, sometimes with friends, and my mom climbs the mountain every year. It's really important to her, and she tries to get everyone up it at least once. Like when I was ten, she got me to the top, but I haven't been able to do it since. The next two years I tried but had to turn back, and then Dad said I had to go to Weight Watchers. But it didn't help—I ended up weighing even more in the end—so now I don't even try to climb."

I blinked back tears, remembering our most recent trip. I had loved it as always, but climbing simply didn't enter the picture, at least not for me. It meant my best friend, Shelly, never climbed either, relegated to the bottom with me. We had fun hanging out and writing and playing cards, but I often suffered twinges of guilt for holding us both back, missing the chance to see Maine again from a mile high.

"Have you tried other things to lose weight?"

"Yeah. I went back to Weight Watchers, but the same thing happened. I lost some, plateaued, then gained it all back. I've also taken iodine to try to improve my thyroid, which didn't do anything. Then when I was fourteen, Mom had me go see a therapist."

Apparently, I didn't do a good job hiding my emotions because Betty looked up sharply from her notes. "Can you tell me more about that?"

I shrugged and played with a strand of hair, trying to be nonchalant. "I guess Mom thought something was really wrong with me, or I had some deep dark secret reason for not losing weight, but the therapist didn't think so. So those visits didn't last long." Inwardly I still seethed. Even one and a half years later I remained resentful and felt betrayed by being forced into counseling. It's why I had refused to cooperate and never gave the counselor anything to work with.

"Oh, and then, since my brother lost a bunch of weight when he went to camp, I kept hoping that when I went to music camp last summer, the same thing would happen to me, but it didn't, even though they have a secondary focus on wellness." Not that my parents had told me about the wellness aspect. No, I found out the hard way when I arrived at camp and had to step on a scale. Not a happy start.

"And is your brother still thin?"

"Yeah, he's on the cross-country ski team, so he eats whatever he wants. That's part of the problem, too." I started playing with a different section of hair. I found it hard to sit without keeping my hands busy. "He eats all kinds of stuff, and so does Dad, and it's fine for them but I'm not supposed to have it, even though Dad's gained a lot of weight, too. He makes all kinds of things, and it's really good because he used to be a professional baker, and it's really hypocritical that he gets to eat it and I don't."

It came out in a rush of pent-up bitterness. I remembered how Dad nonchalantly ate sweets in front of me, and how Mom always bought me sugar-free candy for Easter and Christmas, but Jeremiah got regular candy. I didn't feel comfortable sharing how those things backfired, though, leading me to eat all the forbidden foods in secret.

"Do you think it would be easier if they didn't do that, and that type of food wasn't around?"

"Definitely. And if everyone stopped paying so much attention to what I eat and how much I weigh. It makes me feel like nothing else matters."

I swallowed hard, again on the verge of tears. I remembered all the times I had waited for my parents, especially Dad, to praise me for something, anything—my straight A's, my writing (even if so far I had only collected rejection slips when I tried to publish), my work on the school paper, my flute playing, singing in chorus, my involvement with church. But none of it seemed to matter.

"Is there anything else you'd like to tell me?"

I shook my head. I had already said more than enough.

She nodded and smiled again. "Thank you for telling me all that. I know it might not have been easy, but it was very helpful. Now, this isn't a diet, so I won't be weighing you or telling you what to eat. But I may make suggestions, and I'll meet with you for an hour a week for twelve weeks. I'm also going to meet with your mom for a half-hour a week, to get her thoughts. How does that sound?"

"Good." To my surprise, I meant it. I hadn't realized how nice it would be to simply have someone listen without immediately telling me what to do or that I had something wrong with me. Maybe I could dare to hope, at least a little.

On the way home, Mom asked, "So did Betty have any suggestions for you?"

"Mostly to start paying more attention to what I eat, and why I'm eating it, and also to start doing a little exercise."

I couldn't quite keep from grimacing. I hated pretty much everything about exercise—jiggling, sweating, getting out of breath and red-faced. But I especially hated having anyone else witness such unpleasantness. Thank goodness I didn't have to take gym class anymore.

Mom must have caught my expression. "I know you don't like to exercise." Her tone conveyed how little she understood this, with her fondness for walking, hiking, biking, swimming, ice skating, and cross-country skiing. "So I've been thinking of something that might help. If you exercise for at least half an hour a day, five days a week, after a month I'll buy you a book."

She knew my weakness. The offer didn't make me excited to exercise, but it did make the idea slightly more palatable. "Okay."

Given the rate at which I devoured books, the incentive of one as a reward quickly encouraged me to start using the trampoline or ski machine when I came home from school. Exercising then helped me avoid an audience, since Dad usually napped then, Mom didn't get home until 5:30, and Jeremiah often had after-school activities.

I kept at it, even though the exercise made me pay attention to my body, something I generally tried to avoid, refusing to think it had anything to do with me. I didn't want to notice how much space I took up on the bus seat, practically two-thirds of it, or the effort it took me to climb stairs at school, especially with all my books, or the way food always seemed to fall on the shelf-like protrusion of my breasts when I ate. I knew losing weight would help, but it didn't make me automatically like the process.

I also tried to cut back on sweets, but somehow it didn't work as well. Whenever Dad made something, it seemed to call out to me, begging to be eaten. I didn't know what to do about it.

Then one day after a session with Betty, Mom said to Dad at dinner, "Erik, Betty wants you to come with me at our next meeting on February 10."

Dad did not look pleased. "Why?"

"To see how you feel about the program and to learn a little about your eating style."

Dad glanced down at his butter and syrup-laden French toast, his unease almost palpable. I focused on my own plate, not wanting them to see my gleeful delight. Finally, he would know the discomfort of having someone else scrutinize his food choices!

When the day arrived, I couldn't wait to see his reaction to the visit. I didn't expect him to be happy, but I also didn't think he'd be quite so upset. He stormed into the house, radiating anger, and went right to the bedroom. Then Mom came in with a smile.

I looked at her in confusion. "What's going on?"

"When Betty asked what food groups your father didn't like, he said olives and beer. Then she asked him what he had for breakfast, and he said a chocolate muffin." Mom laughed.

"But we don't have any chocolate muffins, only chocolate cupcakes." Then it dawned on me. "That's what he had for breakfast?"

Mom nodded and laughed again, seemingly unable to help herself. "But he neglected to tell her the 'muffin' had frosting and sprinkles!"

I joined her in laughter. Trust Dad to have a breakfast for champions. "Do you think he'll go back?"

She sobered then and shook her head. "No, he already he said he wouldn't. But I think it helped to have gone at least once."

Somewhat vindicated by this example of hypocrisy, I hoped the experience would make Dad more sympathetic to my attempts. It didn't.

Still, I continued exercising and started paying attention to my food choices. I even lost a few pounds, and on March 9, Mom came home and said, "I think this was the one you wanted."

She handed me my reward for consistent exercise, the book *Arrows of the Queen* by Mercedes Lackey. "Yes!" I grabbed it eagerly, excited to read more about Valdemar and pleased at my progress.

Then on March 23, my meeting with Betty took an unexpected direction when she asked, "Did anything happen when you were a child to make you afraid of boys?"

The first thing I remembered couldn't be considered part of "childhood," at least to me, but still, it rose up, clear and vivid.

It happened on a chilly fall day in 1988 when I took our dog Alaski for a walk. We lived in a rural neighborhood but hadn't had any problems for years. It never occurred to me to worry about going out by myself, at age twelve, especially with the dog.

Until, on our way home, two boys a little older than me stopped their bikes right in my path. "Hey, wanna fuck?" one of them said, leering.

I froze. We stood on the side of the road, no houses in sight, no traffic. Panic spread through me like ice, holding me still. Then Alaski, always protective of women and children in general and me specifically, started barking and lunging at them.

I had never been more grateful for his presence. I wished I could simply turn him loose, but I knew I couldn't encourage his behavior, since we'd already had a couple of close calls with biting.

"Alaski, down." I pulled half-heartedly on his leash.

The boy laughed. "I guess not. The dog wouldn't like it. Maybe another time." They rode off, still laughing.

I finished the walk blindly, badly shaken. I decided to forget about it, choosing not to tell my parents. It meant when they had Alaski put to sleep a few months later because of his aggression, I could only explain part of my grief, the sorrow and anger for the loss of my beloved dog who had only been trying to protect his family. I couldn't tell them how vulnerable I now felt, or why I stopped taking walks for a long time.

But since I didn't consider the incident part of childhood, I started to shake my head in answer to Betty's question. Then another memory came up, this one long-ignored. I didn't particularly want to discuss it, but I didn't know how to say that, or even if she would accept refusal.

"In kindergarten, during recess one day, some boys tried to get me to pull down my underwear so they could look. But I didn't. Instead I kept asking why I should until the bell rang." I rushed through the description, embarrassed.

"Do you think that has anything to do with your weight?"

The question confused me. "No. I never think about it. I practically forgot it happened."

She nodded but didn't seem convinced. "Sometimes things like that can influence us without our being aware of it."

I started getting angry. It reminded me of the therapist. I wanted her to drop it, so I simply stared without saying anything.

Eventually Betty asked, "How have you been doing overall?"

Changing the subject didn't decrease my annoyance. The tone of the meeting became strained, and I left feeling worse than I had going in. I hoped for a quiet car ride home, but Mom wanted to talk.

"Do you remember that incident in kindergarten, with the boys who cornered you?" she asked.

I looked at her, amazed at the coincidence. "I do, but only because Betty asked about it today. I hadn't thought about it in years. That's so strange that you brought it up, too."

"Actually, I mentioned it to her. I hoped she'd talk to you about it."

My anger returned and redoubled. I couldn't even speak at first, afraid of what I might say, furious at being manipulated. "Why?" I asked, finally.

She glanced over at me before turning back to driving. "I was worried you might have been impacted more than we knew, and you might be using your weight as protection."

"Well, it didn't, and I don't," I snapped.

After that I continued with Shapedown because I knew Mom had spent quite a bit of money on it. But any desire to make it work vanished, as did my hope.

22

2 Stealth Eating

Spring and Summer 1992—age 16, 200 pounds

April 2, 1992 (written in a journal I kept for my English class)

I want to write about paganism and goddess-based religions because today, a group of women in Massachusetts are going to perform a memorial for all the women who died in the witch trials.

For the past two years, I've slowly been becoming aware of the goddess religion. When I was younger, I knew nothing about it, and I simply believed in God. (Can you picture me believing in such a figure?) I really had no choice in the matter; I went to a Catholic church until I was seven, and I didn't question things nearly as much then. I was a blind follower. Scary, huh? But then we left that church and started going to Unitarian Universalist (UU), churches, which is where we are now.

Anyway, two years ago Mom started finally asking questions about the Catholic religion, and as a result, I began to be curious about different things. I saw books like When God Was a Woman, Beyond Power, *and* Drawing Down the Moon *around the house, and I started asking my own questions. I began to discover things, and then I saw the films "Goddess Remembered" and "The Burning Times" and I felt my heart break at seeing how much abuse women had suffered at the hands of religion, the tortures and torments of the Crusade and the witch hunts and so much more.*

Of course, I don't believe in a goddess—or any deity—as such, but I do agree with many of the principles. In fact, my church supports the majority of these beliefs; equality, justice, and belief in truth. Also, the "worth and dignity of each individual human being". So yeah, I guess I fit the concept of a pagan. "One who is of the earth." (That's the literal meaning.)

Dad was making chocolate chip cookies. I knew this but tried to ignore it as I packed for a sleepover at Shelly's. But even in my bedroom, well away from the kitchen, the imagined scent of fresh cookie dough made my mouth water. I could picture Dad stirring the chocolate chips into the caramel-colored batter of eggs, flour, butter, sugar, vanilla, baking soda. I could almost taste the sweetness and feel the crunch of the chocolate. I swallowed hard and tried to focus.

By the time I went into the kitchen to put my shoes on, Dad had started spooning the mixture onto cookie sheets. I knew they wouldn't be done before I left, but I wanted one so badly. Then I saw Dad pop a piece of dough in his mouth, his normal habit to "test" it.

I debated asking for my own "test" taste. Even though I no longer felt committed to Shapedown, I still went to the sessions with Betty, and most of the time I tried to eat well in front of my family. But this time I couldn't seem to help myself.

I asked, "Could I have a little dough, since I'm leaving soon?"

Dad glanced at me. "Do you really think you need it?"

Blood rushed to my face. My heart pounded in a mixture of confusion, anger, and shame. He didn't sound accusatory, and maybe he simply meant to remind me of the questions I should be asking myself. The logic sounded good, but I didn't buy it. I felt like he had instantly judged me based on my weight and hunger for cookies and found me wanting. Why, after all, did someone so large as me need yet more fat? The hypocrisy of not acknowledging his own large stomach made my mouth bitter.

I didn't say anything, simply turned and put my shoes and coat on before Mom came in. "All set?" she asked. I nodded, not trusting myself to speak. Once in the car, though, Mom wanted to chat. "You and Shelly must be almost finished your project."

"Yep."

"How do you think your English class will respond to a project about goddess-based religions?"

I shrugged. "They'll probably say it figures. I mean, they already think of us as the resident witches."

I touched the pentacle I wore as a pendant, the symbol of Wicca, a dead give-away for anyone paying attention that I had an interest in less traditional religions. I also knew most people regarded me as a fat band nerd, only worth the time of day if they needed help with their homework. This would at worst simply be icing on the cake of my unpopularity.

"Do you think of yourself as a witch?"

"I don't know. I mean, it's interesting, and a lot of other UUs are pagan, but I don't I believe in all of it. I do like the idea of a goddess, though."

I didn't say I particularly appreciated the idea of a goddess who did not get portrayed as skinny, like Mary, but as someone full-figured, more like me. I couldn't quite wrap my brain around people worshipping a fat woman, but I liked the concept.

I also didn't tell Mom how bitterly ironic I found it that despite her own developing interest in the older religions, which included those heavier women, she still couldn't seem to accept my weight. She might be happy to have a shared interest with me, and she enjoyed hearing about my various activities, but I knew my weight and finding ways to change it were always on her mind.

Luckily, Shelly lived close by so I didn't have to keep up much more conversation with Mom. I escaped into Shelly's house with relief. Everyone in her family carried extra weight, but they didn't make a big deal about it. It also didn't stop them from having lots of snack foods around. Their pre-packaged sweets didn't taste as good as Dad's homemade ones, but I didn't care. In fact, the novelty of them sometimes attracted me more strongly.

"How are you?" Shelly asked as we went to her bedroom.

"Glad to get away from home. Dad's being annoying."

She gave me a sympathetic grin, her face made even prettier by the expression. "I hear ya. Dads are good like that."

"Did I tell you that he's apparently all freaked out about my interest in Wicca?"

"No, why?"

"I guess he thinks I'll start hating men, and turn into some male-bashing feminazi—or at least that's what he told Mom."

She rolled her eyes as she sat on her bed. "Please. That's like the opposite of Wicca."

"I know!" Feeling better with the sympathy, I put my bag down and sat opposite her. "So, do you want to start on the project, or play cards?"

"Let's work on the project, then take a break for cards."

We spent some time going through everything we had, deciding how to organize it, before breaking. As Shelly took out the cards, I said, "I'm going to use the bathroom. I'll be right back."

When I found the bathroom occupied, I wandered into the kitchen while waiting, automatically checking out the goodies. Swiss Rolls, Nutty Bars, Doritos, potato chips, Klondike bars, and in the glass cookie jar, Chips Ahoy.

I paused. Dad's question about needing cookies still stung, but it didn't mean I didn't want a chocolate chip cookie. The Chips Ahoy would be better than nothing. I managed to scarf one down before Shelly's sister came out of the bathroom, and I plotted when I could sneak a Nutty Bar.

Shelly and her family wouldn't care if I had one, but eating sweets in secret had become ingrained in my psyche. I couldn't even imagine having witnesses to my gluttony. I'd feel too ashamed and guilty. Not that eating in secret stopped those feelings.

When I went to the bathroom, I noticed cookie crumbs caught on my shirt and quickly brushed them away, not wanting the reminder of my weakness. Especially since I also couldn't help noticing how large and awkward my body seemed in the small room, my thighs spilling over the edge of the toilet seat. Why had I eaten the cookie? Why couldn't I control myself?

My inner monologue of self-abuse continued when I returned to the bedroom to play cards. Somehow, it didn't stop my plan to grab a Nutty Bar.

Except no matter how many sweets I got, it never seemed like enough. When I went back home, my desire for sugar remained. Over the next few months, as school wrapped up and summer started, I found as many ways to get it as I could.

Now, instead of exercising when I had time alone at home, I went for sweets. While the cookies lasted, I had an easy time, since I could bring one back to my room. As long as I didn't take one of the last few, no one would notice.

But then Dad indulged his baking habit by making a cake. At my first opportunity to eat some, I considered my options. If I cut an obvious piece, everyone would know. And I couldn't carry it as easily as a cookie. Then I had it.

I glanced around once more. No one could see me. I quickly cut a thin sliver all along the edge, so you couldn't tell at a glance it had shrunk. I stuffed the cake in my mouth as fast as possible, barely chewing before I swallowed. Then I washed the knife and my hands, and voila! No one the wiser but me. Plus, I could do the same thing with brownies, although I never quite figured out how to manage pies.

Around the same time I started babysitting for a nearby family. "Help yourself to anything in the kitchen," the parents said. I could hardly believe it. They would give me, a fat girl, free access to their food? Were they crazy?

I couldn't wait for the kids to go to bed to raid the chips and ice cream. Even so, I made sure never to finish anything, and I always scooped out the ice cream to match the existing contours, making my forays less obvious.

But sometimes I craved candy, a little harder to get since I didn't drive. Before school finished, I could sometimes hit the vending machine, using money from babysitting and my allowance. Once summer arrived, though, my options became limited. Which is why, on August 5 when I asked Mom if I could go with her to the mall to visit the bookstore, I had an ulterior motive.

While she went to the grocery store, I first headed to another store to furtively purchase a Snickers and Charleston Chew. My heart hammered the whole time, somehow convinced Mom would see me, or someone else would and tell her.

It distracted me from realizing the major flaw in my plan until too late. I didn't have anywhere to put the candy bars. My pants, already tight, had barely enough give to let me slip some money into the pockets—candy bars certainly wouldn't fit. Since I didn't have a purse, I quickly bundled the bars in my jacket before backtracking to the bookstore, terrified all the while to find Mom already waiting for me.

Only when I didn't see her did I relax and look at the books. The two aisles of sci-fi and fantasy felt familiar and safe, one of the few places where it didn't matter what I looked like. I happily browsed until Mom came to find me.

"All set?" she asked.

I reluctantly put down the next book in the Valdemar series and made sure I had a good grip on my jacket. "Yep."

I kept the candy hidden all the way home, feeling like I had made it safely. Until I realized Mom had followed me to my room.

"Is something wrong with your jacket?" Before I could answer or protest, she sat next to where it lay on my bed and opened it up, exposing those treasured yellow and shiny brown morsels. As I saw them through her eyes, though, they no longer seemed appealing. I grew all too conscious of my weight and bulk, the way the bed creaked when I shifted. She looked at me with terrible disappointment and sighed.

"I knew you had something when you wouldn't put down your jacket. Why did you get them?"

How could I explain to her, whose sole vice seemed to be eating a few chocolate chips from a bag in the cupboard every now and again? (Sometimes the bag moved to my parents' closet, but I always knew where she stored it and when I could safely raid it.) Then my bottled anger boiled up.

"Because I get so tired of everyone focusing on my weight, sometimes it makes me want to eat more."

She fell silent a moment, absently smoothing the sleeve of my jacket. "Do you want to lose weight?" she asked finally.

I flung up my hands in exasperation. Was she kidding? Did I want to get to a point where I didn't breathe hard simply by walking, where I didn't have to worry about people snickering about me behind my back, or fearing what people saw when they looked at me?

"Yes! But I want to do it for my own reasons, not be pushed or manipulated into it."

"I'm sorry if you feel manipulated. I'm worried about your health."

"I know, but I still need my reasons."

"Do you want to see Betty anymore, or maybe that new counselor, Bob?" I felt surprised but pleased she asked.

"Not really."

"Okay." She drew a deep breath. "I'll cancel your appointment, and I won't bring up your weight again unless you ask for my help."

Finally! What a relief. I leaned over to give her a hug. "Thank you."

The next day I had a chance to write about it in my journal.

Well, yesterday I told Mom pretty much how I feel about going to see another counselor, or seeing Betty, or about other people commenting on what I eat. I'm not saying that some of this hasn't helped. It has. I eat more vegetables since starting Shapedown, fewer snacks, I exercise more, I drink more water—but despite all that, I've gained weight because I was so angry I wanted to get revenge.

So now, what am I going to do? I'm gonna try to lose weight in my own way and by my own terms, eating what I want when I want, and not being ashamed about it (at least, that's the theory). As of today, August 6, 1992, I weigh about 200 pounds, and I'm 5' 1". At one time, that would've thoroughly depressed me, but now, I'm still so mad that I hardly care anymore. But I do want to lose weight, as I've said about a google times before (so I exaggerate some). At any rate, by the time I graduate, I'd like to weigh 125 pounds, which means losing 75 pounds in two years. So, wish me luck!

3 Love Feast
August 1992—age 16, 200 pounds

August 1992

Everything about me seems constricted. I want and I ache for so many things, but locked inside this body and this world, I begin to think I can't have them. I want to lose weight, I want to fall in love and get married, I want to write and get published, I want to sing. I want so much! And yet, it really isn't so much if one thinks about it. For at least some of the time, I want to be happy, although now I'm not, not really.

Life here is definitely lacking a certain shine, which is why I so desperately desire change, and even as I wish these things, I work against myself to stop them. I need some inner voice to yell at me when I go wrong, make me remember. I can't do this on my own – I'll admit that, but I don't want outside help. It's so unfair.

I know, I know. Life isn't fair. I'll be the first to say it, but it doesn't mean I have to be happy about it. I'm trapped in a small town world, trying to grow and change when the area and people I'm around won't permit it, even if they aren't aware of that fact. I've got two more years of hell until I get out of high school; how am I to survive? I mean, right now the only reason I'm keeping my sanity is because I'm writing. If I didn't have that, I know I'd flip. And yes, I'm going to Con-Con, so that'll be fun, but still.

"I can't wait to go to Con-Con," I told Shelly during one of our long phone conversations, mentally counting down the days until the third week of August.

"Remind me what that is again?"

"Sorry." I went into my room to talk in relative privacy and flopped onto my bed. "It's the Continental Conference for Young Religious Unitarian Universalists, or YRUUs, so it's easier to say Con-Con, especially since we call the regular conferences cons already. It'll be a big group of us from all over the country, and maybe even Canada. It moves around, but this year it's being held in Poland—Maine, not the country. And Jeremiah and I are getting in for free, since our Senior Youth Group advisors, Paul and Noel, are working at it and we're going to help watch their kids."

"What will it be like?"

"I'm guessing similar to the regional cons, but bigger and with more options. Workshops about different things, exploring spirituality, some time for worship services, music, and probably some people getting fairly touchy-feely."

"Sounds pretty cool."

"Should be. Mostly I want to be out of the house for a while." I sighed heavily. "Every time I start to listen to music, Dad complains that it's too loud, and he's always asking me why I like listening to stuff that sounds so angry."

"I hear ya. My dad's the same way. Clearly they don't understand the appeal of Pearl Jam and Soundgarden."

"Well, maybe that's a good thing. Can you picture our dads headbanging?"

We both laughed. "Good point. But going back to this conference, will there be any cute guys?"

"I'm sure. I mean, if I see cute guys at the cons in Maine, there must be some from around the country." At least, I hoped so. While I knew any boys I liked wouldn't want anything to do with fat me, I could appreciate the view. "Don't worry. I'll take good notes."

I guessed right. I saw plenty of boys I considered cute, mostly ones with long hair, among them our youth leader, who went by the name of Yoda. To me, he looked like a short version of Pearl Jam's Eddie Vedder, which meant I instantly adored him.

But I didn't talk to any of them beyond pleasantries. I wanted to be as cool and carefree as the other teens, who lounged in skimpy clothes, traded massages, and cuddled. I couldn't do it, though. Their lack of self-consciousness only emphasized my body image issues. I watched from the outside, lonely and longing, and angry with myself for not having lost weight sooner. That would have given me the confidence I wanted.

Jeremiah, on the other hand, fit in perfectly. Given his outgoing nature, he mingled and spoke easily with everyone. Plus, although it was weird to think about, objectively I recognized he had become very attractive: lean from cross-country skiing and bike riding, with wavy hair a little past his shoulders, sometimes with an auburn beard, teeth now straight after braces, and green eyes sparkling behind contacts. I could have trailed in his wake, but I had grown tired of only getting sympathy attention as his overweight sister, something I ran into with his friends.

Then at dusk on the second day we had the Love Feast, held by the lake. At first, I stood on the periphery and only observed: the candles winking like fireflies on the picnic tables; the crowds of people milling around in tie-dye and flannel and henna tattoos and long hair and dreadlocks; the trees turning slightly amorphous against the darkening sky; the soft ripple of the water under the chatter; the cool breeze; the first stars beginning to shine; the bowls of finger food on the tables.

Then everyone quieted to listen to Yoda. "The Love Feast is inspired by a story about a group of people who wanted to know what heaven and hell were like, so they went to visit them. In hell, they found everyone seated at a huge table filled with food, but everyone looked hungry. The group realized it was because the table only had very long forks, and people couldn't feed themselves, so they were forced to sit in front of the food without eating.

"Then the group went to heaven. To their surprise, it was almost the same as hell, with the same long table piled with food, and the same long forks. But in heaven, everyone was happy and laughing, because they had learned to feed each other. So tonight, for the Love Feast, you can only eat what other people feed you. And I ask that you feed one another in silence."

Most people immediately grabbed grapes, pretzels, pieces of candy, apple slices, popcorn, and whatever else they could find on the tables before feeding each other, some solemnly, some laughing. But by some unspoken rule, they all hugged after exchanging food.

My heart hammered. Did I dare take part in this? Would anyone actually feed me? Would they recoil if I fed them and offered a hug? Could I even think about this food offering as something done only out of love, not judgment? Did I deserve to be included?

Then one of the girls in my Shamanic workshop came over with a smile and proffered a grape. I felt slightly silly, like a baby, as I opened my mouth and she popped the grape in. It tasted sweet and faintly tart as I chewed. She gave me a quick hug then walked off. As she left, my heart expanded like the Grinch's when he discovered the true meaning of Christmas. With a smile, I grabbed some peanut M&M's and ventured into the crowd.

I looked specifically for Yoda, but I also found others who had been kind to me, and no one turned away from my offer to feed them. Yoda even returned my shy hug.

Then, to my utter astonishment, the leader of my Shamanic workshop approached. He had coffee-colored skin, black hair, and smiling brown eyes; clearly far more attractive than me. Yet he gave me a pretzel, a sweet smile, and, unprompted, enveloped me in a warm, nurturing embrace. I hugged back automatically, hardly knowing what to think. It seemed like he cared about me in some way, that he didn't hug me because of the Love Feast but rather the event gave him an excuse for the hug. He stepped back, gave me one last smile, and disappeared into the crowds.

Overwhelmed, I wandered down to the shore, arms wrapped as far around my middle as they would go. I stared at the gentle water, sparkling with reflected moon and starlight, and then I cried as quietly as possible. I could not remember feeling so accepted and welcomed. I looked down at the few remaining M&M's in my hand and realized for the first time in a long while they didn't tempt me. Hope quickened in me. If I could hold onto this moment, maybe I really could meet my goals and lose weight for myself.

Feeling unexpectedly free, I hushed my breath and wiped my tears as I walked back to the feast. I still didn't have the courage to talk to my workshop leader, but for the rest of the week my heart remained lighter than it had in years.

Not long after, I told Shelly about it while we were ostensibly going to sleep in my bedroom, the night before my family's annual trip to Baxter State Park. I couldn't help smiling in the dark as I spoke, still floating with happiness from Con-Con.

"That's pretty awesome," she said. "And you did get pictures of this guy who looks like Eddie, right?"

"Definitely, along with a lot of other cute guys. Oh, and we played a game where we passed a kiss around in a circle, and I stood between these two tall guys with long hair, so they each kissed me on the cheek and I got to kiss them, although they both had to bend down about a foot."

What a surreal moment, when they had actually played the game and kissed me instead of running away or faking it.

"I'm so jealous! But I'm glad you had fun."

"Me, too." Then I glanced at my clock. "We should probably go to sleep for real this time. It's almost midnight."

We woke early the next morning for the five-hour car ride to Baxter State Park, keeping ourselves entertained on the way with games, conversation, and tapes we'd made of the Dr. Demento show. We arrived and had the lean-tos set up by 2:30, leaving plenty of time to stretch our legs.

"Do you want to go up to the falls?" Jeremiah asked.

Shelly and I looked up from playing cribbage, glanced at each other, then said in unison, "Sure." Grinning, we put on sneakers and headed for the trail.

I'd been to Katahdin Stream Falls before and knew it wouldn't be easy, especially towards the end when we'd have to scramble over steeply inclined bare rock face. A very different mile than what I walked at home. So it didn't surprise me to immediately fall behind Jeremiah and Shelly. Even without a backpack, carrying my heavy body steadily up and over rocks proved incredibly hard, no matter how slowly I went.

When I paused to catch my breath, I had a moment of deep bitterness. Why had I been so lazy? Why hadn't I gotten my act together to lose weight?

Those questions plagued me every year at Baxter. Most times, they reduced me to tears and despair. Often they made me push too hard in an attempt to prove, at least to myself, that my weight didn't keep me from being capable.

Then I remembered Con-Con, how accepted I had felt. Maybe this time I could accept myself and my limitations. I decided to try that novel approach. Instead of attempting to keep up, I allowed myself to go at my own pace. It didn't make the hike easy, but it did become more bearable.

When I arrived at the top of the falls, breathing hard but at least not feeling like I might die, I found Jeremiah and Shelly waiting. "Everything okay?" Shelly asked.

I looked at the gorgeous falls tumbling over root and rock. It all looked so much more beautiful than when I forced myself to hike too fast, and my already happy heart raised another level. I smiled. "Yep, everything is great."

Late August 1992:

When we left Baxter, I knew I'd miss it. Even after Mr. Spastic Squirrel woke me up at 5:30, and the sun wouldn't let me fall back asleep, I'd miss it. I'd miss the wide open expanse of sky, the majestic sweep of the mountains across the horizon, the chatter of the animals, the carefree camaraderie of being with other people who love nature, the way the water rippled over the rocks, the way the animals weren't afraid and didn't have to be. In such a place, in the glory of it all, one's heart sings, one's soul lifts, one discovers oneself. No matter the inconveniences, that feeling cannot be found elsewhere, where one sits and stares in awe of creation, reveling in one's part in this great fabric of unspoiled nature, no matter how big or small, for all is beautiful, as it was intended.

4 He Likes Me! But Why?

Fall 1992 to Summer 1993—age 16–17, 200 pounds and gaining

Fall 1992

Recently, I've been thinking a lot about my emotional state, and I realized that I haven't been this happy since 8th grade. And it's very odd. I didn't expect to be happy. But school's not bad, class-wise (administration still sucks, but hey), and the discovery that I'm not alone, that I have two friends who feel like soul-sisters, gives me enormous strength. That helps so much. Each day, it's as though a part of my soul that was torn and bleeding heals up a little each time people I like return the favor. It's the most incredible feeling. I'm discovering myself, I think.

I read back on things I wrote last year, and it's so lost, "desolate" as Shelly put it. I had no hope of improvement in the near future—it simply didn't seem possible. But now—things are different. I didn't know who I was, and while I'm still not entirely certain, I believe I have a much clearer sense of self than I had. I am much more comfortable with my being because I am finally coming to terms with aspects of myself that I had never before acknowledged simply because they were degraded by much of society, even sometimes my family.

I wondered at times if my happiness could last, but mostly I tried to simply accept it. In addition to spending time with friends, going to concerts, writing, reading, playing in band and taking flute lessons, I had a new project: helping with the school newspaper. Jeremiah had become editor, and we had far too much fun putting in subversive articles and cartoons.

I didn't think things could get any better until I found out I'd be attending another big conference that fall.

"I got selected as a delegate for the YRUU United Nations Disarmament Conference. I'm going to New York on November 19!" I told Shelly.

"Cool. Is that the one Jeremiah went to last year?"

"Yeah, and he had a great time."

I didn't add that she had hit on part of my excitement: in this, at least, I was my brother's equal. Nor did I pause to think much about the reality. Of course Jeremiah, a thin extrovert, would love going to the biggest city on the East Coast and meeting lots of new people. The fact that it might be different for me, a fat introvert, didn't completely register until I left.

My parents dropped me off at the Portland Jetport. "Call us when you get there," Mom said, giving me a hug.

When I exchanged hugs with Dad, he gave an unexpected piece of parting advice. "Have a good time, and watch out for boys."

I didn't know if he meant it as a warning, or he wanted me to be on the lookout for anyone eligible. I had the sense he sometimes worried when I didn't display much interest in boys my age, at least around him. My idolization of long-haired rock stars and actors, whose posters plastered my bedroom walls, didn't impress him.

I didn't have much time to think about it, because once they left, I immediately felt overwhelmed and out of place as I contemplated flying for the first time, all alone. The airport seemed far too big. I became abruptly self-conscious about my appearance. What had I been thinking, going out in a skirt showing my bare, thick calves, and the fat of my upper arms trying to burst from the confines of my short sleeves?

Panicky, I went to the bathroom, hoping for some semblance of privacy so I could get myself together. That backfired when I unthinkingly looked in the mirror, something I generally avoided. Any previous embarrassment paled in comparison to this newly discovered horror.

I had a double chin.

A slight one, to be sure, but visible. I stumbled back to the gate and numbly followed others onto the plane. Even the tightness of the seat and seatbelt trying to contain my wide hips and protruding stomach barely registered. When had I gotten this fat? Having my weight so prominent and visible in my face seemed somehow worse than anything else.

Then shock turned to anger and disappointment with myself. Why couldn't I have even a shred of self-control and willpower about food? Why hadn't I been able to get in better shape over the last few months, when everything else was going so well?

I realized I'd grown complacent, assumed the pounds would miraculously fall off once life improved. Now I knew, too late, it didn't work that way. Instead of being excited about the conference, I became abruptly scared and sick at heart.

My anxiety only increased when I arrived in New York. The crowds and my uncertainty about where to go left me feeling six instead of sixteen. I nearly cried. Desperate but obstinate, I refused to ask for help. I dreaded judgment in someone else's eyes saying of course I would be useless and lost and stupid because of my weight. Instead I wandered, vaguely going where I thought the instructions said, hoping by some miracle I would end up in the right place.

"Hey Erica!"

Could someone possibly be addressing me? I craned my head around and saw someone waving.

"Over here!" a girl I'd met at Con-Con said.

Her smile saved me, and I even managed one in return as I joined her and a small group of other youth. Maybe I would survive after all.

Once at the hostel, as I met the youth delegates from the other districts, I couldn't help remembering Dad's parting comment. Initially I didn't think he had anything to worry about, or get excited about, depending. Not that the boys looked bad, just too preppy for me.

Then a latecomer dashed in, wearing sandals and baggy red tunic with a rope for a belt, with wavy, light brown shoulder-length hair. I admired him from a distance and heard someone call out, "Chris!" It made me smile even more, since a couple of years before I'd had a huge crush on another Chris. The name seemed like a good omen.

Still, I had no expectations or delusions about his interest in me. To my astonishment, as we gathered to hear a speaker from Nigeria in the evening, he sat next to me on the floor. "Cool braids."

My fingers, busy putting little braids into my long hair, stopped momentarily. "Thanks." I wondered if I had wandered into a parallel universe. Why else would he be talking to me?

"Mine aren't that good. I never get them quite tight enough."

I picked up on his Southern drawl. It made him even more appealing. "You know how to braid?"

"Yep. My name's Chris, by the way." He held out his hand.

I shook it dazedly. "Erica. Nice to meet you."

"You, too." Then he grinned, eyes twinkling mischievously. "Do you mind being my pillow?"

"Um, okay."

He stretched out and put his head on my thigh. "Ah, much better."

A cute UU my age who knew how to braid, had a great accent and long hair, who not only didn't run away but actively suggested physical contact? I was lost.

Hence my dismay when, despite having spent much of our free time together over the few days of the conference, he only wrote back to me once after I returned home.

"That sucks." Shelly's assessment matched my own.

"Yeah, but maybe it's for the best. I have plenty of other stuff to think about."

"What do you mean?"

"Well, Mom's having a tough time with a couple of her kids. Who knew third graders could be suicidal or super aggressive? So I'm helping her grade papers, especially math and spelling. And I really need to focus on school, since Jeremiah's Valedictorian and I want to try for that, too. Then Jeremiah and I are trying to get a concert together as a fundraiser for the school paper—which, by the way, will be awesome if it happens."

"I know. I really hope it works out!"

"So do I. But then, Jeremiah will be gone next year, and it's going to be so strange being alone with my parents."

"I know what you mean about older siblings leaving, although at least I still have a younger sister around. It definitely changes the dynamic."

My concern grew in early 1993, when Jeremiah became increasingly absent as he left for college visits and a trip to Hungary with his English class. Sometimes I saw him only when working on the school paper. At least we had the concert as hoped, and everyone loved it.

Then the letter Jeremiah received from Northeastern University changed everything, although at the time I didn't know quite how much.

"You're not going to believe this," he said after reading it.

"What is it?" Mom glanced over from making a salad.

"I got accepted, but that's not all. They're offering me the full academic scholarship they told me about."

"Really?" Both Mom and Dad spoke at once before hurrying over.

Sure enough, based on his class rank and SAT scores, the school offered him a free ride. Jeremiah wanted to go to Cornell, but the money won out.

No one said it, but I sensed the increased pressure of matching Jeremiah's academics. After all, my parents didn't have any money for school, so scholarships were our best bet. I didn't like it, but a fierce sense of competition, as well as my own desire for academic success, saw me through junior year with straight A's.

By the time summer rolled around, I hadn't exactly forgotten about Chris, but I didn't think much about him, either. Which is why I was confused one evening when Dad said, "There's a young man on the phone for you."

I took the phone. "Hello?"

"Hey, honey, it's Chris. I'm at Ferry Beach for a UU retreat for the week and thought we could get together."

The months of silence vanished. He wanted to see me! He called me honey! Of course I agreed.

I went to Ferry Beach the next day, excited and nervous. Would he still want to be seen with me? Would we have as much fun as in New York?

My nervousness turned to something like dismay when I saw him. He had shaved his hair except for a long swath down the middle, a wilted Mohawk falling over one side of his head. My heart sank further when I started talking to him. His ready smile and twinkling gaze had vanished, replaced by a more typical teenage sullenness.

The visit passed slowly, brief conversation punctuated with awkward silence. Part of me simply grew resigned. What more could I expect? I had a keen awareness of how much space I took up on the couch, how much heavier I was than anyone else at the conference. Who would want to be with me?

Then hope rekindled when he asked, "Could I come visit you for a day or two?"

"Sure, that would be great!"

I hoped a change in scenery would help, and at first it did. Once at my house, he smiled more and became physically affectionate, putting his arm around me and giving me hugs. He continued to use endearment terms like honey, and he even consented to the somewhat awkward process of posing while Dad took pictures of us.

It gave me enough hope that I tried not to be visibly upset when our conversation went in directions I didn't like or expect, which happened with alarming regularity.

In late afternoon we went for a walk, and when I told him about my love of fantasy books, he replied, "Those aren't really any better than Harlequins."

Crushed, I changed the subject by saying, "And see that house? I used to get horseback riding lessons there."

He didn't even acknowledge what I'd said. "I need to pee. I'll be right back." And he dashed into the woods.

I tried to figure out some way to salvage this, even though he clearly wasn't following the script I had created in my head. What could I do to get his interest, to have him be engaged in the conversation? Maybe I needed to lighten up.

So I tried to make a joke of it when Chris came back and said, "I think the only way people can really get to know each other is to have sex."

"Really? So everyone has to be bisexual, then?" He didn't laugh.

It still didn't prepare me for his behavior later in the evening. Sitting next to me on my bed, he asked, "Have you ever been kissed?"

I didn't think the couple of pecks on the cheek during the game at Con-Con counted. "No."

He moved fast. Despite my open bedroom door, his tongue went down my throat, and one of his hands went up my shirt while the other roamed more freely. I froze. I had no idea what to do. I had hoped for a kiss, but not like this. My first kiss expectations had all been set by Disney and romantic comedies, something sweet and tender. This struck me as demanding and fierce, almost threatening. Relief swept through me when Dad opened a nearby door, startling Chris into jumping back and shortly after leaving my room.

I stayed awake for a long time, trying to calm down and make sense of what had happened. Should I say something about it? But what? How could I protest after the fact when I couldn't in the moment?

The next morning Chris acted like nothing had happened, so I did, too. I wasn't sorry when he left, nor surprised I never heard from him again. In retrospect, it seemed he thought he could take advantage of me, due to my size and obvious low self-esteem. Why had I imagined he might be interested in me as a person? It made me furious at him, and at myself for being so vulnerable.

I didn't feel comfortable telling my parents about it, but I needed to tell someone. I ended up talking to Jeremiah, and he commented, "That asshole."

His supportive anger helped a little, but not enough. I couldn't put it out of my mind for a long time. I didn't like Chris's behavior, yet part of me believed I should have expected it. I should have known better than to think a boy would actually care about me, to see beneath my weight to my inner self. Much as I longed for that, I did not, after all, live in a romantic comedy or fairy tale. And if I didn't feel like my own father could be proud of me as I was, and focus on things other than my weight, how could I expect it of anyone else?

Part of me rebelled against the thought. I was miserable about my body but also determined to be recognized as more than that, even if it meant pushing the point further. The end result? I gained more weight.

5 Comparisons

Fall 1993 to Fall 1994—age 17–18, 230 pounds and gaining

September 10, 1993

I want to go hide in a corner somewhere where no one can see me. It's better not to be seen than to be seen and not noticed. So many people ask me how Jeremiah's doing, ignoring me, that I feel like some sort of messenger. That's part of why I'm somewhat loath to even try going to Northeastern. It's as though, if I'm in a place where he is or has been, we're constantly going to be compared, and I'll be the one lacking. Jeremiah's smarter than me, better looking than me, more talented, easier with people, and far more charismatic and amusing. After seeing him, why should anyone care for me?

Oddly enough, though, this doesn't make me jealous, make me hate him. I'm envious to be sure, and I think he's incredibly lucky, but I've grown resigned to it. I've gotten to accept the fact that I'm not particularly gifted or unique—though others may tell me otherwise, it's not enough. I don't feel like people should remember me—I'm always surprised if people know my name.

The day I found out my class ranking—Valedictorian—did not go quite as I'd hoped.

I had rarely been so ecstatic. I had done it! I had lived up to my brother's example. Walking to class felt more like floating. I didn't even notice how much space I took up or the effort of climbing the stairs. When I walked into my Physics classroom and heard everyone talking about class position, trying to figure out who ranked number one, I smiled. I couldn't wait to tell them.

"Mike, are you Valedictorian?" someone asked.

He shook his head. "No, I'm Salutatorian."

"Sheila?"

"I'm third. Maybe it's Shelly?"

"Not me. I'm fourth."

Then our teacher came and started class, but I could hardly pay attention. I instantly deflated. No one had asked me. No one had even glanced my way except for Shelly. Maybe they would have asked had the conversation gone on longer, but I doubted it. Their avoidance struck me as something deliberate, as if they didn't think a fat person could possibly be smart enough to achieve such a status.

Only when class finished, as we packed up our books, did Shelly ask, "Erica, what rank are you?"

By then I almost didn't want to answer but said, "First."

"Congratulations!"

No one else said much to me. I went through the rest of the day trying not to care what anyone else said or thought, but it didn't stop my misery.

My excitement stirred again on my way home. Surely Mom and Dad would be happy. And as soon as I told them, Mom gave me a huge smile and hug. "Congratulations! I'm so proud of you."

My glow of pleasure lasted until Dad said, "Excellent! Now you need to apply to Northeastern and see if you can get the same scholarship as Jeremiah."

Not a word of praise or acknowledgment from him. It felt, again, that the only way he would ever tell me "I'm proud of you" would be if I lost weight. Until then, nothing else truly mattered, except now maybe I'd get some money thrown my way. My happiness at my grades melted into bitterness, particularly when he brought up Northeastern.

I wanted to argue, but the practical side of my brain kept my mouth shut. Not only would the scholarship guarantee a free education, but with Northeastern's co-op program I'd have the added bonus of valuable work experience and earning money. So I applied. It didn't make me happy about it.

"I hope I don't get the scholarship," I told Shelly one afternoon as we played cards at her kitchen table. I knew I sounded whiny and ungrateful, but I couldn't seem to help it.

"Why?"

"Because if I get it, I feel like I won't have a choice about where to go. It's not as if my parents have any money to help me out."

"Yeah, I know the feeling."

"And I know in one way it'd be awesome not to have any school debt, but I *really* don't want to live in Boston for five years. It's too many people and not enough nature."

"Maybe it won't be so bad." I just looked at her. "Okay, yeah, it might suck. But you can always come visit me at Bates when it gets too bad."

I smiled wanly. "I'm sure I'll take you up on that."

Her words reminded me of something else I had been trying to ignore. Whether I went to Northeastern or not, everything would soon change. This familiar ritual of playing cards in her kitchen would become nothing more than a memory. We wouldn't have sleepovers anymore, finish each other's sentences, laugh when teaching French to fourth-graders, or go to concerts together.

Thinking about it depressed me sometimes to the point of tears. I could hardly imagine what it would be like not to see Shelly every day. We had been friends for ten years, and shared all the same classes for the last five, and nearly everything else in our lives. She had been my only consistently close friend in all that time, and now the only one left at all. Who would I talk to once we went our separate ways?

I reminded myself we would stay in touch, and, after all, I had made friends at music camp. Surely I would be able to find some kindred spirits at college, though I suspected I'd have an easier time if I went to my first choice: Tufts, with its Universalist heritage and pretty campus outside the city.

I tried harder to convince myself Northeastern would limit their scholarship to one student in a family, or at least one at a time. But I didn't truly believe it. So when my offer letter came, I reacted only with sinking resignation, not surprise and certainly no joy.

Besides, after Jeremiah's scholarship, my offer seemed anticlimactic. As with my Valedictorian status, my parents' pleasure looked more like vindication, not a celebration of my achievements. Not that I blamed them. I, too, did not believe I had accomplished anything special, since Jeremiah had done it first.

I didn't want to go and live with strangers in a city where I wouldn't be able to see the stars at night or be close to forests, but my pragmatic side won out. I accepted the scholarship, and in September 1994 I moved to Boston.

Despite my trepidation, I tried to convince myself it wouldn't be too awful. It didn't work. What I didn't expect was how bad it would get.

6 Judgments
Fall 1994 to Fall 1995—age 18–19, 240 pounds

January 14, 1995

Have you ever been in pain, pain that is ever-present, continual, that seeps through you and stabs into you every day, every minute, maybe every second, and if you move to make it better it only sends fresh waves of agony, lapping over and over, wearing down the stones of your resistance, until you can do nothing but sit and cry? I do not mean emotional pain, or at least not at first—that is something we all feel. No, I mean physical pain, pain that becomes as much a part of you as breathing, awareness of which never leaves you until you can no longer remember what it was like to live without it.

Two months of never-ending pain, of fear, of anger, of loneliness. I know what it is like now, and I have become adept at dealing with it, at sponging away blood, at taping on bandages, at clenching my teeth tightly when the pain comes so the only sound I make is a small gasp. Oh, yes, I am now wise in these ways—but what I would not give to have remained ignorant.

When I first moved to Northeastern, I had mixed feelings. As a freshman, I had to stay in a dorm, but my scholarship meant I could live in Kennedy, the Honors Dorm. Only when I saw it did I realize how much of an improvement it offered over the standard freshmen dorms that had small bedrooms and communal bathrooms.

"This looks nice," Mom said when we found my suite on the third floor of Kennedy.

I nodded, looking around curiously to take in the small living room, bathroom, and two bedrooms. One bedroom, quite small, had bunk beds in addition to two desks, but my bedroom had enough space for both beds to be on the floor. Relief washed through me. I didn't even want to think about the possibility of having to struggle up to a top bunk.

My roommate had already moved in, but she said, "Are you okay with that bed? We can switch if you want."

I smiled, pleased at her friendliness, although I could tell from her slim build, designer clothes, make-up, carefully arranged hair, and boy band posters that we had little in common. "No, this is fine, thanks."

My parents helped me bring up all my stuff, and then we headed out, planning to stop by Jeremiah's place before they went home. As we left my room, a young woman with a blonde ponytail and glasses poked her head out from a nearby door. "You must be new. I'm Janice, your RA." At my blank look, she said, "Resident Assistant. I'm here to help out if you need anything or have questions."

"Nice to meet you. I'm Erica Bartlett."

Her face broke into a wide grin. "You must be Jeremiah's little sister!"

I groaned inwardly. I had gotten all through high school without people calling me that, and it didn't seem fair to have it crop up in college. But I only said, "That's me. We're actually going over to see him now."

"Say hi to him for me, and I hope you'll come to Honors Tea sometime."

"Honors tea?"

"Every Thursday some of us get together at the Honors Lounge for tea and munchies."

"Okay, I'll think about it."

As my parents and I walked over to Willis Hall, where Jeremiah shared an apartment-style dorm with three other guys, I started noticing all the differences from home. The busy streets with aggressive drivers, rows of buildings all close together, the lack of greenery, crowds of people, all the pigeons, and the sheer cacophony. I also couldn't help realizing how much space I took up on the sidewalks, how out of breath I became even on the short walk. My shoulders tensed, and I wondered again what I had gotten into.

My concern only increased over the first month. No one said anything about my weight, but I keenly felt the effort of taking stairs when the elevator in my dorm went on the fritz (an unfortunately common occurrence), as well as my tiredness from all the walking, the sense of shame as I squeezed between the arms of a seat in one of the large lecture halls, or tried to walk behind a row of chairs at a table to get to an empty seat. I decided to arrive early at class when possible so I could sit at the end of the row.

My self-consciousness kept me from talking much with my classmates, particularly since many of them seemed to be hard-core computer geeks, having built their own computers and already done some programming, much more than my limited experience with the school newspaper, video games, and LOGO. I did start getting friendly with one of the other girls in my dorm room, and I met a few more people at the Honors Lounge.

"This is Erica, Jeremiah's little sister," Janice said when she introduced me to people.

Part of me resented not having my own identity, but another part appreciated the connection, since it gave me a small sense of belonging. Even though Jeremiah had started his first three-month co-op job for civil engineering and couldn't go to the lounge for tea, my designation as his little sister stuck.

Having those few connections also meant I didn't have to sit by myself when I went to the cafeteria. I sometimes sat with my roommate, or Janice, or another girl named Sarah from the honors dorm, an engineering major who had hair even longer than mine, falling in a long trailing braid down her back.

"I never realized how spoiled I was by the food at home," I said early on, not quite sure what to make of the options in the cafeteria.

"What do you mean?" Janice asked.

"I'm used to vegetables from the garden, for one, and to my dad making everything from scratch." I picked up the pallid, pasty pink slice on top of my turkey sandwich. "They call this a tomato?"

"Good point. It doesn't look much more alive than my chicken patty." Janice poked experimentally at the frozen and reheated brown disc on her plate. "At least it's not moving."

I did like one thing about eating at the cafeteria: no one policed my intake of sweets. Having chips, donuts, cookies, or ice cream in front of other people still embarrassed me, but at least it couldn't get back to my parents.

I appreciated the liberation, especially since I sought comfort in food as a way to cope with all the change. Even academics, easy enough through most of high school, now made me struggle. I had never been around so many people as smart as me, or smarter. I had the same experience with band, playing with musicians who actually cared about music and practiced voluntarily. I became all too familiar with the sense of being a tiny fish in a very big pond, making everything harder than expected.

But those complaints all got blown out of the water in mid-October, when I stepped out of the shower, glanced in the mirror, and froze when I saw a lump on my chest.

Centered right between the tops of my breasts, no bigger than a pea, hard to the touch but at least not painful. Still, it didn't seem like anything good. Not quite sure what to do, I followed my preferred method of treatment: I ignored the problem, hoping it would go away. Instead, the lump grew with frightening rapidity to the size of an apricot.

My mind raced with panicked thoughts of cancer until I went home for Columbus Day weekend and my family doctor diagnosed it as an infected cyst. Unfortunately, the antibiotics he prescribed did nothing for it, so I went to Northeastern's health center at the end of the month. They took one look and sent me to a hospital to have the cyst drained.

I dreaded both the concept of surgery and the necessity of meeting a new doctor. I suspected my weight would inevitably come up. I only hoped the discussion wouldn't be too awful.

My hope shriveled into dust beneath the cold, calculating gaze of the man who would operate on me. I could see my size reflected in his eyes, the sheer amount of space I took up on the exam table, and I read judgment on his face before he asked, "How long have you been obese?"

Even though he hadn't said a word about my cyst, I clearly felt his implication: my weight, and nothing else, had caused this problem. I yearned to make some sharp retort, no matter how banal, but scared and in pain and self-conscious in the stupid white johnny, I quailed and simply answered the question.

"Since I hit puberty."

I could feel his disdain and disgust as he prepped for surgery. Only a huge effort of will kept me from crying. But the tears came later, as I lay alone in the hospital after being cut open by someone I knew held me in utter contempt. It felt like the night would never end.

My sole satisfaction came the next day when I returned to my dorm room and called Mom to tell her what had happened. She exploded. "That bastard!" Since she almost never swore, somehow this cheered me. "Will you be okay?"

"I think so, but I have to change the dressing while the incision heals, and I'm not looking forward to that."

I didn't elaborate. I didn't want her to worry, but more, I preferred not to focus on the details of how deep the incision went, of packing and unpacking gauze in the gaping hole. I had never been bothered by blood, but bandaging my own wounds tested my resolve. I dealt with it by simply making it part of a new routine, knowing I had little other choice.

Needing to change the dressing made me grateful all over again that I didn't have to use a communal bathroom. I couldn't imagine trying to deal with this without some level of privacy. At the same time, my illness isolated me. I didn't know anyone well enough to share my experience and simply suffered in silence. At least I had always been a morning person, and the other three got up later than me. It gave me the necessary time to change the bandage, trying not to think about what I had to do even while looking for new places to put the medical tape, which constantly irritated my skin.

After a couple of weeks I got tired of doing it and went to the health center to have them change the bandages. Having someone else pull and add gauze felt worse than doing it myself, though at least they gave me some hypoallergenic tape to use. I decided to just take care of it myself from then on. I stuck with my plan until one morning not long after when I noticed something new.

The horrible stench of infection.

I knew it too well from when my uncle had been in a motorcycle accident and had his leg amputated after infection slowly, insidiously crept up from his mangled foot. Smelling it in relation to myself sent me into a terrified panic. I raced to the health center, and they immediately sent me back to the doctor who had done my surgery.

"You have a staph infection." He looked at me with renewed disgust. "You're not keeping it clean enough, so you'll need to use alcohol pads and take antibiotics."

I felt humiliated and furious anew. I understood exactly what he meant. Clearly, because of my weight, I must also be unhygienic. Never mind the fact that staph infections mostly happened in hospitals. I wished I had the courage to tell him to go to hell, but again, I meekly took the judgment and prescription.

Even more frustrating—and frightening—the infection refused to go away. It showed up as lesions on random parts of my body, the inflamed red spots growing and sometimes bursting, resulting in the need for more bandages. The lesions disappeared when I went on antibiotics but came back as soon as I stopped. The antibiotics themselves gave me a topical yeast infection on my chest, making my skin red and stretched-looking. My body seemed to be falling apart.

In desperation, I went to another doctor, this time a dermatologist, hoping for some relief. Another vain hope.

He gave me a patronizing smile. "The lesions could be from your clothes being too tight and rubbing against your skin. I think we should focus on shrinking you." He made a slenderizing motion with his hands, as if I needed the clarification.

I wanted to rage at him, to yell, "I've been overweight for years and this never happened—that's not the problem!" Instead, I smiled through gritted teeth, left, and never went back.

I reserved my energy for staying afloat in classes, trying to keep my grades up, and getting through the holidays without revealing how much I hurt, how simple movements became agony. I hated even thinking about being an object of pity.

Finally, around New Year's, Mom told me, "Dr. Lindsey thinks you should start taking Echinacea to boost your immune system so you can finally kick this infection."

With nothing to lose, I gave the Echinacea a try. It worked like magic. I found it ironic that of all the people I had seen, my chiropractor proved the most helpful. But I didn't care where the help came from. I was simply relieved by the end of January to feel human and pain-free again, an almost forgotten sensation.

But the damage had been done. I now carried a multitude of scars from the cyst and the results of the staph infection, making me, if possible, even more body-conscious than I had been. The incision from the cyst healed but didn't close completely, leaving a small hole right between my breasts, making the whole thing worse.

At least in January turtlenecks, long sleeves, and covered legs didn't seem unusual. I did my best to refocus and get back to a normal life.

Seeing Jeremiah more often helped. After finishing his three months of co-op, he returned to classes for three months, and to our amusement, we ended up in the same Calculus 4 class. Our professor gave us a strange look but mostly seemed relieved to learn we got along.

Being in classes also meant Jeremiah had more flexibility in his schedule. It allowed him and his roommates to hold a party for a marathon viewing of the *Star Wars* trilogy to show off Jeremiah's new subwoofer.

"And we're going to play a *Star Wars* drinking game," he said when everyone arrived.

"Um, really?" I didn't drink, but I couldn't help glancing at Janice, wondering how a bunch of underage students would pull that off with an RA present.

She saw my expression and laughed. "None of us are drinking alcohol, but we have milk, soda, water, and juice, so pick your beverage. But pace yourself, because it's a lot of drinking."

I looked at the rules and saw what she meant. It included items like: "Drink whenever Yoda talks like a fortune cookie. Drink whenever Darth Vader sees one of his children and doesn't recognize them, twice if he tries to kill them. Drink every time someone gets a hand chopped off." We wouldn't quite be drinking every minute, but not far from it.

We only got through *The Empire Strikes Back*, but I laughed more than I had in a long time. Even better, laughing no longer hurt. I went back to my dorm, still grinning.

My reclaimed life lasted until mid-February, when Jeremiah told me his new girlfriend, Natalie, was pregnant. "So I think I'm going to need your help getting through Calculus 4," he added.

"Okay. I'll do what I can." I didn't quite know what else to say.

Jeremiah and Natalie got engaged not long after, and from that point on, almost everything outside of classes revolved around the wedding and coming baby. Amidst the whirlwind, I did experience one side benefit: as my parents focused more on Jeremiah and less on me, my relationship with them improved. Having a bit of distance between us didn't hurt, either.

Natalie, now part of the family, came on our trip to Baxter State Park in the summer. She hiked up to Katahdin Stream Falls with us, and I hated that she had an easier time than I did, even at seven months pregnant.

Angry with myself all over again about my weight, I pushed hard, trying to keep up, until my face turned red and I couldn't hear anything over my pounding heart and fast breathing.

I found Dad waiting at the base of the falls. He took one look at me and said sharply, "You need to stop and rest."

His concern only made things worse. I didn't want him to witness this proof of my inability, of how my weight crippled me, to give him an excuse to say he was right. I found I wanted to just go home. The park had failed to offer its usual comfort.

Although still not happy about going back to Boston, I did look forward to being an aunt, and I wasn't disappointed when my niece, Marie, came into the world not long afterward. When I held her for the first time, looking at the perfection of fingers and toes and ears and eyelids and silky skin, I wanted to cry. I had been like this once, too, a little cherubic being. How had I grown so monstrous and flawed? Yet despite my double chin, enormous chest and stomach, and multitude of scars, as soon as I held her, she gave a little contented sigh, snuggled against me, and relaxed.

Blinking back tears, I smiled down at Marie, amazed this tiny human being had accepted me so completely and instantly. If only everyone could treat me that way, with no judgment. And if only I could treat myself that way. Maybe I could learn something from her.

7 Cookies to the Rescue

March 1996 to August 1996—age 19–20, 240 pounds

"Building the Cage", Part 3 of a story called "The Road to Freedom", written March 1996

Does everyone hate themselves? I wish I knew, because then I'd know if what I'm feeling is normal or not. Hah. Who am I kidding. Nothing and nobody is normal. It's just an ideal invented by psychiatrists and social workers that no one can achieve, so therefore everyone has problems and has to go see one of these "professionals" for help. It's such a scam. But there I go again, avoiding the issue. Yet one more item for my list of Why I Hate Myself. Let's see what we have so far: I'm fat, I'm ugly, I don't have any friends, I'm boring (hence the previous item), I'm insecure, I lie to myself, and (now) I avoid confrontations.

God, I wish I just had the guts to kill myself and get it over with. But I can't even do that because in the back of my mind there's this stupid, irrational little voice that keeps saying, "It'll get better. Life will improve." Like hell. The only way it'll improve is if I remove myself from it. I can't even stand to look in a mirror, I'm so disgusting. At least if I killed myself, I'd be doing everyone else a favor. They wouldn't have to look at me all day long. I'm surprised I don't make anyone ill.

I furtively wiped at my tears as the words poured out. For the first time I appreciated the cave-like environment at work, lit only by the glow of computer screens since the guys refused to turn the lights on. Then again, had I been working elsewhere, someplace where they let me have light, at least during lunch so I could read, or where they offered to help me learn my job, I might not be writing this.

Where did I go wrong? I was so adorable as a child. What did I do to deserve this transformation from beauty to beast? I really wonder why I bother. No one is going to answer my questions.

I think, if I weren't so gross, I'd be an actress; I'm already so good at pretending. Fulfilling that stupid myth that fat people are jolly, like Santa Claus. Only Santa Claus doesn't exist, and how should I be jolly when people call me a cow, or porky, or say I'm dull?

I'm not dull; I'm actually too sharp. I've cut myself open inside with my razor edges, but as the wounds are internal, no one notices. It's only a matter of time before I drown, the blood from these wounds pooling into my lungs. There are a few small channels that might carry away the pain, but already I am walling them off. People hurt too much. I don't want to ever get close again.

Not that getting close to people seemed to be an option here. I thought back to the fall of 1995, not long after Marie's birth, when I had started the process of getting my first cooperative education job in the computer science field.

Along with the other sophomores planning to start co-op during the first three months of 1996, I attended a bunch of meetings with our co-op advisor, who talked about resumes, references, and interviews. I half-listened but mostly hunched over my notebook, doodling and trying not to panic. My resume, at least, had something going for it, but how could I attend an interview and promote myself when my self-confidence verged on the negative?

Going shopping with Mom one weekend for a professional outfit only emphasized my concerns. Time after time I'd try something on and she'd ask, "How does it fit?"

"It's too tight," I inevitably said, or, "The top fits but not the bottom," or "I can't zip it up all the way."

By the time I found a dress at Fashion Bug, I wanted to crawl under a rock and cry. Mom didn't help when she asked, "Have you thought about trying to lose weight again?"

I laughed bitterly to keep back the tears. "Of course I have, but I only have so many food options on campus." I thought of the chicken tenders and curly fries at Chicken Lou's, my forays to Burger King and Pizza Hut, and my modest attempt at healthy eating by getting occasional salads.

"And I've told you about my roommates and their kitchen habits. It doesn't exactly make me want to cook." I shuddered even in memory. As a sophomore, I now lived in Willis Hall, sharing an apartment with three older students, none of whom did dishes on a regular basis. One had even left a half-eaten pot of pasta on the stove for a week. "It's not as if I'm happy about this either, you know."

Thankfully she let it drop, and I returned to Northeastern, armed with my one outfit and resume. I interviewed at two defense contract companies, and even though I made the cardinal mistake of emphasizing my lack of experience, both surprised me by offering me jobs.

"Which one did you take?" Mom asked when I called to tell my parents.

"The one at Draper, doing IT support."

"What made you choose that?" Dad asked, one of the few times he chimed in. Normally he let Mom do all the talking.

"It's closer, for one, so I can still get back in time for band and even do orchestra. It also has really good benefits, including vacation time, and good pay, and I feel better not writing software for any potential military use."

True enough, but those were only secondary reasons. I couldn't quite say how when I heard the specifics of the other job, and how much the people there expected me to easily pick up programming, I quailed, suffocated by the fear of failing and disappointing them. Much easier to not even try.

And yet, I had stumbled badly even with this safer job. Over two months into my co-op at Draper, I didn't have much more ability to fix computers than on my first day. Talk about a failure.

I didn't truly realize how depressed I had become until I looked at my story on the screen. I hadn't planned to write anything autobiographical, but this had some truth to it, particularly when I considered my adolescent years. I knew I had friends, and some people cared about me, but it wasn't always easy to remember.

I took advantage of those raw emotions, turning what I had written into part three of an eight-part prose piece called "The Road to Freedom," a story about a girl like me who eventually found her way out of pain and isolation to become the person she was always meant to be.

I hoped to use the piece as inspiration on discovering my own path to the same end. It didn't work.

Having roommates who all smoked only made things worse, since it largely left me to hide in the bedroom, the one smoke-free room. When I had gone home for the holidays and told Shelly about the housing situation, she asked, "And they didn't let you change apartments, even though you asked for a non-smoking room?"

I flushed in embarrassment. The thought of trying to change rooms had not occurred to me. I assumed I simply had to deal with it. "Well, I didn't ask."

"You still could."

I thought about trying to move while starting co-op in winter and not knowing whom I'd end up with. Maybe it would be even worse. "I've kind of gotten used to it. I mostly stay in the bedroom, and I'll be working a lot, so I'll manage for now."

I didn't tell her, or anyone, about the new problems when I started my job.

My body self-consciousness had increased to the point where I didn't feel comfortable showing an inch of skin beyond face and hands, no matter how hot the rooms at work became from all the computers. The other co-op students largely ignored me, leaving me feeling useless and ashamed.

I only had a few bright spots in my days: band, orchestra, my writing, visiting with Jeremiah, Natalie, and Marie, and the prospect of going to Baxter State Park. Despite the disastrous hike the year before, I needed time at the park to get away from all the people and computers and smoke and life. Sometimes it seemed like the only thing keeping me going, even with the trip still months away.

Happily, some improvements came my way. In the last month of my co-op, not long after my meltdown while writing "The Road to Freedom," someone finally started showing me the basics of how to fix computers, and one of the staff members enlisted my help with a project.

When I left at the end of March, I had at least done something. Encouraged, I decided to go back for my six-month co-op over the summer and fall in an attempt to redeem myself.

I also got excited when my three months of classes started up again and a friend called to ask, "Did you know Northeastern is opening a grocery store on campus, and we can use our Husky Money there?"

Like me, she had a full scholarship, which meant each school quarter we received Husky Money to spend on campus. "No, I didn't. That's great!"

"And I thought it would be fun to do some more cooking, but I don't know a lot about it. Do you want to come over here sometime and experiment?" She had lucked out with housing and had a single.

Get out of my smoky apartment, dirty kitchen, and eat some real food? "I'd love to!"

Not everything went smoothly. For instance, we tried quesadillas with avocados, except I'd never had an avocado and didn't know how to pick a ripe fruit. The rock-hard one I bought didn't work so well. But we had some success, and visiting and trying new things gave me something else to look forward to.

The best change, though, came shortly before returning to work at the end of June when the smokers all moved out. I had a notice about getting new roommates, but to my utter delight, by early July, "No one has moved in!" I enthused to Mom over the phone.

"Does that mean you have the apartment to yourself?"

"Yes." My mouth hurt from smiling so widely. "So I'm airing everything out and burning candles to get rid of the smoke smell, and now I can do some more cooking and baking."

"That's wonderful!"

I agreed, but I couldn't quite tell her the best part. Living by myself for the first time was miraculously freeing. No one watched what I did or ate. To my surprise, I ate better and even started exercising of my own free will in the apartment, where no one else would see me jiggle and sweat. I didn't have a scale, so I couldn't tell if I lost weight, but I did have more energy.

The icing on the cake came with changes in the co-op situation. Another girl joined us for the summer, one with a strong will who refused to work in the dark. Simply having some light proved a huge relief and made the office more comfortable.

The real shift, though, came in late July when I brought in chocolate chip cookies made the way I'd learned from Dad.

One student absently ate a cookie, but in short order he came back for another, then another. "These are awesome!" he exclaimed. "Do you have some secret ingredient?"

"No, just my dad's recipe."

I couldn't help smiling at his response. He had been the one to first start showing me around, and between that, his blue eyes, blond tousled hair, rugged good looks, and ready grin, I had a definite crush. I didn't plan to do anything about it—apart from my own issues of insecurity and body image, his fondness for guns and limited interest in reading gave me pause—but it still made me happy seeing how much he liked my baking.

Word spread, and soon a little group huddled around the container of fast-disappearing cookies. "Oh my God, these are heavenly!" the head of our department said, her expression blissful as she carefully caught each crumb.

I hadn't expected such an enthusiastic response, and after that, things only got better. My confidence improved when interacting with others, knowing I could do something they liked, and it also seemed to me they reciprocated by treating me with greater consideration. My involvement with fixing computers and other projects increased.

For the first time I discovered the joy of feeding others. Seeing how much people enjoyed the sweets gave me almost as much pleasure as eating them myself. I continued bringing in treats—brownies, cake, pie, and more—but everyone agreed the cookies were the best.

By the time I went to Baxter in August, I felt better than I had in a long time, physically and emotionally. It allowed me to do the hike to Katahdin Stream Falls much more easily than the year before, a further confidence boost.

Meanwhile, Mom and my eight-year-old cousin made the trek to Chimney Pond—3.3 miles each way—and when we regrouped in the evening, my cousin couldn't stop talking about the hike, enthusiasm shining in his eyes.

"It was so awesome! I got to climb all over these great rocks, and we saw a snake, and the mountain is so big!"

I laughed despite being envious, especially when I later saw photos. The pond looked incredibly beautiful and peaceful, surrounded on three sides by glacier-carved mountain ridges, water rippling in a gentle breeze. Considering how much easier the hike to the falls was than the year before, I made a decision: the next summer, I would get to Chimney Pond, no matter what.

8 Chimney Pond

August 1997—age 21, 240 pounds

May 10, 1997

It's strange; here I was, thinking up questions to ask Shelly about the whole study abroad experience, and I find myself suddenly getting excited. I know it's still a few months off, but already I am starting to think this is going to be one of the pivotal times of my life.

And there are other things that I am excited about doing before I get to England. I am looking forward to going to Baxter and climbing up to Chimney Pond. I will be glad to go home for Memorial Day weekend and see Shelly and everyone else, and just be in Maine for a while. I am dreading/anticipating the end of the month when I will know for sure if the short stories I submitted to magazines were accepted or not.

So suddenly, it seems I have a lot to look forward to, but I am also finding I regret that I didn't try to get in shape so that this year I might climb all of Katahdin again, not just part of it.

I hadn't told anyone about my obsession to get to Chimney Pond. It therefore came as a surprise to Mom when, at the start of our trip to Baxter State Park in August 1997, a year after her hike with my cousin, I said, "I'd like to go to Chimney Pond."

"Really?" She looked at me in pleased amazement.

"Yep."

The idea made me nervous and excited. Nervous because I had stopped exercising the previous fall as soon as my new roommates, all field hockey players, moved in. Their athleticism made me self-conscious again about huffing and puffing in front of them. But I didn't let my lack of preparation stop me. Having made my decision the year before, I had to do the hike. Envisioning success kept me excited and motivated.

Then I glanced at Shelly. "Are you game?"

"Definitely."

The next morning, though, I wondered if we'd even start. When I first woke up, heavy rain drummed on our lean-to, and I felt cheated. After deciding to climb, I couldn't believe the weather might prevent me from attempting the hike. To my relief, the skies cleared by 10:45. Everyone scrambled to put on hiking boots and backpacks then we headed out at 11.

"Why don't we let them go ahead," I said to Shelly, gesturing to the larger group of Mom, Dad, Jeremiah, Natalie, and Marie in a baby backpack. "We can talk more and take our time."

"Sounds good. You must be excited about England!"

"Very!" I would be leaving mid-September for a three-month study abroad in London. "It'll be so cool to live in another country for a while."

"And at least you speak the language." Shelly had enjoyed her semester in Greece the previous year, despite a language mishap when, after misreading labels, she once used salt instead of sugar when making French toast.

"Yeah, that's a definite bonus."

We talked easily for a time, since the first part of the trail had only a modest incline. The path didn't have many rocks or roots, the surrounding trees gave shade and coverage from any last sprinkles, Roaring Brook's rushing waters sounded soothing in the background, and everything sparkled after the rain. The idyllic setting helped me relax, and my confidence inched up.

But forty-five minutes later the path grew steeper and had bigger rocks, giving me my first real test. I immediately fell behind Shelly. As I lifted my legs higher and higher, then stepped up onto the rocks, my thigh muscles protested. We had moved away from the brook, and without the sounds of water my increasingly labored breathing rang loud in my ears. The beauty around me had not changed, but I no longer noticed it. I remembered how hard climbing seemed to my ten-year-old-self, but I would have given almost anything to have that lighter body now, not this behemoth.

Before long I gasped, "Can we—stop—for a—minute?"

Shelly, only a little winded, nodded. "Sure."

I sat on a rock, grateful for its cool dampness as heat radiated through me. I wondered if I had gone crazy. Did I really want to do this? Would it be worth it? For inspiration, I pictured the images I had seen of the pond, but I needed more. I focused on my desire to prove I could do this, refusing to be stuck at the bottom of the mountain any longer. It drove me on.

"Let's go," I said, not quite ready but not wanting to lose my determination.

After another hour of struggle, the trail briefly leveled, and the trees parted enough to get a view of the mountain's summit. My spirits lifted slightly. Then we saw a sign for a viewpoint and followed the narrow, winding path to a clearing where the world opened before us.

"Oh, wow," Shelly and I said in unison.

We stood on a small section of level ground, dotted with gnarled, wind-twisted trees and a few rocks, surrounded by gorgeous views. Katahdin rose majestically to our left, while to our right we could see the landscape below and how far we'd come. The sky showed no signs of the earlier rain, and the brisk wind revived me.

"It's amazing." I smiled at everything. This is why I had come.

We stayed long enough for a good rest before pressing on. The respite energized me enough to keep going, but afterward I hated nearly every minute of the climb. My will battled my body and gravity, somehow moving me up and over every incline, no matter how steep. My legs turned to jelly, my hair started escaping its braid and sticking to my face and neck, my lungs continually screamed for more air, and my heart sometimes seemed like it might burst.

More insidious was the despair. At the bottom of each rise, I fought back tears, feeling like a failure, hating myself for being in such an unfit state. Sometimes only the sight of another hiker started me moving again; I didn't want any witnesses to my anguish. And each time I'd find Shelly looking rested and eager as she waited for me.

When we hit the level patch leading to the Chimney Pond campground four hours after starting out, fatigue trumped my excitement. Grateful I didn't have to lift my legs very high anymore, I didn't care how I must have looked with my pants half-ridden up my calves, my face patchy with red splotches, and my T-shirt soaked and sticking to me.

"You made it!" I looked up to find Mom beaming at us as she and the rest of my family came our way. "We were just starting to wonder."

I noticed how fresh and relaxed she appeared, though she now carried Marie in the baby backpack. But Dad didn't look happy, and Jeremiah and Natalie seemed frazzled. I wondered what Shelly and I had missed.

"How long have you guys been here?"

"About an hour and a half. We need to head down, but let's get a group picture first."

We all crowded around the Chimney Pond sign proclaiming we had made it up the 3.3 miles. Exhausted, I forced a smile. Once Mom and the others started down, Shelly and I walked through the campground to the pond itself.

The view humbled me. The clear water moved gently in the breeze, reflecting back the glacier-carved bowl holding it, sides of the mountain sloping away with stunning beauty. Sunlight flickered and shimmered on the rippling pond, with the sky a piercing blue overhead. My heart overflowed.

"What do you think?" I asked Shelly with a big smile.

"It's awesome! I'm so glad we came, and I'm proud of you for making it."

"Thanks. Me, too."

I sighed with contentment, relieved and also proud of my accomplishment. Apart from my first time up the mountain, I had never done anything so strenuous, and for the first time I had a vague idea of why people pushed themselves physically. Maybe this meant one day—and not so far away—I could stand again atop Baxter Peak.

The good feeling lasted until we headed back to Roaring Brook and our lean-to. At the first decline, I tripped and fell heavily. "Are you okay?" Shelly asked.

Shaken, I assessed the damage. "I think so."

I didn't get quite so lucky with my next fall. "I think I twisted my ankle."

Shelly tripped right after I said it. "Ugh—so did I," she gasped.

We pressed on, and by the end my legs could barely hold me upright. We limped into the ranger's station at 7:20 that evening, and then to our lean-to, where I collapsed.

Shelly had enough energy left to fetch water for us to clean up. Washing and putting on fresh clothes helped, although I discovered some spectacular bruises in the process. Once clean we hobbled to the other lean-to for dinner.

Everyone applauded when we showed up, and two-year-old Marie ran over with what seemed like an obscene amount of energy. "Ecka!" she exclaimed, throwing her arms out.

I leaned down for a hug. "Hey, kiddo. I love you, but I really need to sit down."

We went to the picnic table, and my appetite returned with a vengeance at the sight and smell of burgers, hot dogs, cut up cucumbers and tomatoes, Doritos, and Dad's famous chocolate chip cookies. I devoured more than seemed possible while listening to everyone else talk about their day.

"Your father got muscle spasms at Chimney Pond and was rolling around on the ground, clutching his leg and saying, 'Ow, ow'!" Mom said with a mischievous smile.

Jeremiah picked up the story. "Marie thought it was a game and started imitating him. It was really funny."

"Oh, yeah, real funny," Dad said huffily. "Don't forget you got muscle spasms, too."

"Is that why you were carrying Marie on the way down?" I asked Mom.

"Well, that and Natalie twisted an ankle."

"Yeah, me, too," I said.

After Shelly and I told them about our descent, Mom asked me, "So are you still glad you went?"

"Yeah, and next year, I want to do it again but be in better shape."

I said this with a great deal of conviction, before I discovered I couldn't even climb the stairs to my second-floor apartment at school, which lasted for a full two weeks. That alone might not have dissuaded me, but I simply had no way of knowing the next summer would bring much greater challenges.

9 Catalyst

July 25, 1998

So here I am, doing my best to help everyone, and I'm wondering who's supposed to be helping me. I'm laying here crying because I'm scared. I'm so scared to see Mom after her surgery, to help her change bandages, to see her helpless and not in control. She always has been the strong one in the family, and it's not fair that she's the one to be struck with this. I'm well aware that life isn't fair, but I can't help feeling angry about it.

It had started the evening of July 13, 1998, while I sat on my bed, doing cross-stitch, watching *Babylon 5,* and generally feeling okay about life. I'd finished a great junior year—including my trip to England, where I made a couple of new friends from Ireland and Belgium, and a week sailing trip on a schooner—while Jeremiah had graduated and landed a job at a Boston civil engineering firm.

I finally had my own bedroom in a new apartment at Northeastern, I had enrolled in a correspondence writing course with the Institute of Children's Literature, and I had just started my final six-month co-op at Draper Labs in Cambridge. I had even come up with a plan (again) to lose weight. Admittedly, the apartment had mice, one of my roommates drove me nuts, and I'd suffered some emotional ups and downs, but overall everything seemed fairly settled for a change.

Then I got a phone call from Mom. "Erica, I have some bad news. You know how I told you I was getting a biopsy? The results came in, and it turns out I have breast cancer."

I fell against the wall in shock. Mom climbed mountains and went on bike races, ate lots of fruits, and mostly stuck to vegetables she grew herself. How could she have cancer? But she did. All the certainty in my world crumbled away.

"How bad is it?" I asked.

"We're not sure yet. I'm going to have a mastectomy and reconstruction at the beginning of August, and they'll check my lymph nodes then. From what we can tell so far it seems pretty contained. I'll start chemotherapy in the fall, and then maybe radiation in the spring, depending on what they find."

Chemo. My hand reached to touch my long hair, a lighter version of Mom's pride and joy. Losing a breast and her hair would be incredibly hard for her. I tried to ignore the ache in my stomach as I wondered what this would really mean. Would Dad be a good caregiver? What if something went wrong? How would I react to seeing Mom like that?

We talked a little longer, but I couldn't absorb the details. I barely slept, and the next day I went to work unfocused and frightened.

Everyone tried to be supportive, telling me, "She'll be fine," and, "Breast cancer is one of the most treatable forms of cancer."

I swallowed down screams. I didn't want reassurances for something with no guarantee. I wanted someone to acknowledge it was okay for me to feel scared and sick at heart. But no one did, at work or elsewhere.

For added pressure, when I talked to Jeremiah about it, he said, "You're the most level-headed person I know, and I think you're going to be the one to get the family through this."

I didn't disagree, but I didn't want the responsibility. That had always been Mom's job. At the same time, what choice did I have?

At least Mom found a little humor in the situation. "You won't believe this," she told me a few days later. "The doctor says I need to gain weight!"

We laughed at the irony. "Why?" I asked.

"Since they're using my stomach fat and skin for the reconstruction, they need about five more pounds to work with, so I'm eating lots of potato chips and your father's goodies."

"Too bad I can't give you some of my fat."

"I asked, but apparently they haven't figured that out yet."

Her ability to still laugh gave me needed courage to go home and stay for a few days after her surgery to help out. It seemed surreal for her not to be able to tie her own shoelaces, or even sit up from the couch, without a helping hand. Yet she handled it with patient grace, at least around me, giving me some peace of mind.

But I found it hard to grasp when she said we would still go to Baxter just a few weeks later. "Are you sure?"

"Absolutely." Her tone left no room for argument.

We arrived at the park without incident, although driving along the miles of bumpy dirt road brought her a lot of pain. She didn't complain, just clutched a pillow hard across her half-healed stomach. And in an unusual twist, she stayed at the bottom of the mountain while Shelly and I went up to the viewpoint along the Chimney Pond trail for lunch.

I did a little better on the hike than the prior year. It helped to know we weren't going as far and could take a lot of time. Seeing the sign for the viewpoint still relieved me, knowing we could turn around after our lunch.

When we entered the clearing, I paused to take in the stunning panorama of sky, mountains, lakes, and trees. Then reality hit me. "This is so strange."

"What?"

"I can hike more than Mom." I wiped my eyes, barely able to get out the words. "It's not supposed to work that way."

Shelly gave me a hug. "I know."

Despite my sorrow, I managed to enjoy Baxter, finding it restful after the hectic pace of the city. It gave me enough of a breather to gather some strength for what I knew would be coming.

I went back to Boston, and Mom started chemo, losing hair and energy. Living away from home meant I had limited awareness of the impact on her, and I suspect that's what she wanted, so I could finish school without getting too derailed by concern.

It worked, and as she approached the end of chemo treatments in March, I looked forward to an uneventful last quarter of school. I had also made my schedule light, taking only three classes, one of those being Piano. I wanted to finish with as little stress as possible.

The easy schedule turned out to be a good thing because Jeremiah and Natalie separated in March, and Jeremiah ended up with custody of Marie. My limited classes allowed me to help bring Marie to daycare a couple of days a week. Then, after I graduated, the three of us moved back to Maine and tried to pick up the pieces of our lives.

July 11, 1999

Some part of me has not quite come to grasp the fact that I am truly living in Maine for the rest of my life. But now that I am mostly recovered from the last leg of school, I intend to use this new opportunity to reclaim some of what I lost or didn't appreciate from my youth.

I also must keep reminding myself of Mom and her health. Though she is doing well now and regaining her strength, in the backs of all our minds is the knowledge that she could be dead in five years from a recurrence. If that happens, I do not want her to be worried about me. I want her to see me happy for once, and so I am going to make a very concentrated effort to get in shape.

And there really are things that I would like to do again that I cannot do unless I am in better shape. I dearly want to climb Katahdin again, to be able to go up stairs without gasping for breath, to go canoeing, swimming, cross-country skiing, ice skating, and horseback riding. I want to be able to do active things with Marie, and be comfortable enough with my body to wear a bathing suit in front of strangers. And it would be extremely wonderful to be able to buy clothes more easily.

And so my task is to draw strength from this land, to let it into my soul despite the barriers I raised as self-preservation in Boston, and I mostly must remember why I want to do this: to feel better, to be able to do more, to make sure that no one has cause to worry for my health in the coming years, to be strong because if there is one thing the past year has taught us it is that we do not know what trials we will face, and we must be ready for anything.

Mom, at least, had become more like her old self by then, back to gardening and walking and some biking. Not needing a wig anymore made her ecstatic, even if her hair had more gray and had oddly become curly. She had enough energy now to get excited on July 23 when a software company in Portland offered me a job doing customer support.

She gave me a big hug. "That's wonderful news!"

"Thanks." I smiled back, happy and relieved.

The job, good to have in and of itself, also meant I could move out of the house. I couldn't wait. It had been suffocating living at home again after five years on my own.

I found a nice apartment in Portland on a bus route. Taking the bus instead of driving gave me extra time for reading and writing. As an added bonus, Shelly lived about a mile and a half away, since she had started attending the nearby University of Maine law school.

Jeremiah also landed back on his feet, finding a job in Gray and an apartment in Lewiston, living near to our aunt Patrice and uncle Marcel so they could help with Marie.

Life seemed to be improving. I liked my new job, where I learned to provide customer support for the software my company designed. The people I worked with were nice, and I enjoyed both my autonomy and the paycheck.

Even so, going to Baxter State Park in August once again came as a huge relief. So many things had changed over the past year, and I had barely had time to pause and absorb it. Sitting on the rocks by Sandy Stream Pond, one of my favorite spots, I relaxed a little, letting the constancy of Katahdin and its surroundings soothe me, give me a sense of stability.

Our second evening there, Dad told Jeremiah and me about the idea he had for Mom's Christmas present. "It's a panoramic photo from the top of Katahdin, and you can even see the curvature of the earth. It's pricey, though, so I wondered if you two would contribute towards it."

"I'm in," Jeremiah said.

"Me, too," I happily agreed. Even with Christmas a long ways off, it sounded like the perfect gift.

After returning from Baxter, life resumed its new routine, but unfortunately it didn't last. Mom's health declined again, starting with low energy and then trouble breathing, to the point where she stopped teaching and often tethered herself to a portable oxygen tank. We didn't know what caused the problems, though, until December 14.

She called me at work. "Can you come over for dinner? There's something I need to tell you."

Abruptly terrified, part of me wanted to protest and run the opposite direction. I knew it couldn't be good news. Maybe if I didn't hear it, it wouldn't be real. But I couldn't be so cowardly.

Mouth dry, I managed an, "Okay."

She broke the news after dinner. "The cancer came back. It's in my liver and both my lungs."

My heart pounded. "But you could get more chemo or radiation, right?"

"I might be able to get some experimental treatment at Dana Farber, but we don't know yet."

She must have rehearsed it. She sounded so calm, and she didn't look sick. How could this be happening? Crying, I gave her a desperate hug, afraid the moment marked the beginning of the end.

The next ten days passed in a slow-motion nightmare. I stayed in regular contact with Mom and Dad by phone, e-mail, and occasional visits, and even at a distance, the horror of Mom's rapid loss of health and general weakening became only too obvious.

Christmas morning tasted more bitter than sweet. Mom could only watch from the loveseat while I filled her usual role of handing out presents. Marie brightened things some with her enthusiastic response to her dollhouse and her Woody doll from *Toy Story*, but the rest of us had a hard time maintaining our spirits.

After I had handed out the gifts from under the tree, Dad told Mom, "There's one more special present, but you need to close your eyes." Mom obliged, and he went to get the picture from Katahdin. When he returned and had it facing her, he said, "You can open them now."

She gasped. "Oh, Erik," she whispered, tears in her eyes. "Thank you."

"It's from the kids, too," he said, voice uncharacteristically gruff.

We all stared at the gorgeous panorama for a minute, the beautiful primal colors, the gently curving horizon rolling away from Baxter Peak. But I also struggled against the knowledge, held in my deepest heart, that Mom would never again get any closer than this to Baxter State Park or Katahdin.

On January 1, 2000, Mom went into the hospital, and she never came out. She died on January 9, a day after turning forty-eight, while Dad and I watched helplessly, flinching with each of her struggling breaths, not knowing which would be her last, wondering if Jeremiah would make it in time. He didn't.

When it was over, Dad went to get a nurse, leaving me briefly alone with Mom. I couldn't bring myself to look at her now-empty form, ghost-like in the white hospital gown and with half-open eyes staring glassily back. Instead, with grief blurring my vision, I turned to the walls, where the staff had let us put up whatever we wanted for decoration. Countless cards from students, teachers, church members, family, and friends. A painting of turtles by an artist friend. The photo from Katahdin.

Anguish slammed into me as I stared at the mountain. I started crying in earnest. Grief flooded over me, but it went deeper. I had always intended to climb the mountain again with Mom, and now I never would. I knew instantly I would carry that regret with me the rest of my life.

Pain and sorrow fueled my determination, again, to lose weight and get to the top of Katahdin, but initially I couldn't do anything about it. As before, I took on more family responsibility, helping Dad with all the details of the death: getting in the obituary, picking out a casket and arranging a viewing, organizing a Catholic funeral for Mom's side of the family, holding a UU memorial service in April for the rest of us, trying to adjust to the reality of a world without my mother.

Somehow, I muddled through, and by May, while I didn't feel happy, I had moved through my immediate grief. I vowed to focus on losing weight and getting in better shape. I weighed myself for the first time in months, wanting to know my starting point.

The scale read 259, twenty pounds heavier than I'd been at Northeastern.

Sickened, I asked myself: How could this have happened? As soon as I posed the question, the answer came. I hadn't changed my diet, which meant I ate some fruits and vegetables but also a lot of junk food and some take-out. Unlike in Boston, though, I no longer walked everywhere to burn it off.

I started paying more attention to food and exercise, but with no real consistency. Then my birthday arrived.

May 28, 2000

I am 24 today. It is strange knowing that Mom was my age when I was born, and she only lived twice again that long. Given how quickly my 24 years have gone, it is sobering to consider the possibility of only living another 24.

So I've started exercising more, in particular going for walks in the nearby Evergreen Cemetery. It's a huge place—it has street names!— and it's very lovely and peaceful; it's impossible to tell I'm in a city. It's therefore a very nice place to walk for a mile or two. Plus there's a duck pond, and it's where Gov. Baxter's headstone is, which always reminds me of his gift to the state of Baxter State Park, so I think it's appropriate.

I had expected the possibility of already being halfway through my life to motivate me more, but it didn't. Mom's loss still seemed too surreal. I sometimes felt like I would turn a corner into an alternate world where she hadn't died. It didn't help that though we'd held services, we hadn't done anything with Mom's remains, waiting to inter her ashes until the end of August, when friends from Montreal could attend. But it meant I didn't have a true sense of closure.

Then in July 2000, a small, somber group of us went to Baxter: Dad, Jeremiah, Marie, my mom's sister Annette, and me.

Even though Annette had been closer to Mom than either of her other sisters, she surprised us by wanting to come. Annette had little interest in doing without showers, electricity, or running water. She joined us only because she knew how important the park and mountain had been to Mom.

"But please tell me there will be coffee," Annette said.

I laughed, appreciating the brief moment of levity. "Yes, Dad and Jeremiah need coffee, too, and they have a grinder that works off a car battery, so it will even be freshly ground coffee."

"Thank God. I think I'm going to need a lot of it."

The morning after our arrival, we went early to the Big Rock viewpoint at Sandy Stream Pond, taking in the very image we had chosen for Mom's headstone. We got lucky and had the spot to ourselves. The sun sparkled across the water, and the mountain glowed. All was hushed and quiet. To me, it seemed as holy as any church.

Dad pulled out a plastic film canister with some of Mom's ashes, and we gathered around. "Today we are scattering the ashes of Polly Bartlett. She loved this place so much, and I can't imagine her not being a part of it." He glanced at us. "Do you want to add anything?"

We shook our heads. I couldn't speak. Dad emptied the container, and the ashes settled by the base of the rock.

The finality of it struck me. Mom's whole being—her years as a mother and wife, teaching, working with the church and a local land trust, climbing Katahdin—all reduced to these gray specks. Those few remains didn't seem like enough for someone who had lived so large.

Taking in the view, I wondered how many more years Mom would have climbed the mountain given the chance. Twenty? Thirty?

Then the question changed in my mind. What about me? Would I climb Katahdin again? And if so, when?

The thoughts churning since Mom's death, and even more since my birthday, took on an abrupt visceral reality. Looking at Katahdin, I knew in my blood and bones, not just my head, it would be here for ages yet to come. But I wouldn't. I didn't know how much time I had left. Was I, like Mom had been, at the midpoint of my life? Would it all be a slow fall from here? What if I was already falling and didn't know it?

I drew a deep breath. Something inside me shifted irrevocably. I would not give regret a second chance. I would lose weight and climb to that height again, and soon, within a few years. I didn't feel it as a promise to myself, only a simple fact.

As we prepared to head back to the lean-to, Dad said, "Erica, before we have the burial, I'm going to set aside another of these film canisters with ashes for Jeremiah to take up the mountain and scatter. Do you want one, too?"

Had he asked me even an hour before, I'm not sure what I would have said. But now I didn't hesitate. "Yes, please do." I knew without any doubt I would get Mom's ashes to the summit where they belonged.

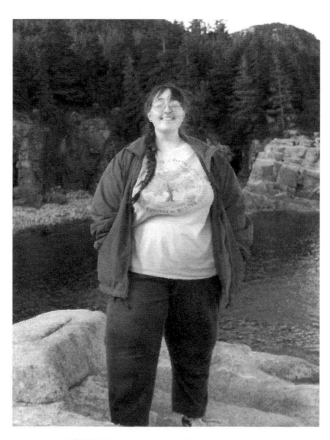

Fall 2000, Erica at Acadia National Park

Part 2 I'm Shrinking!

10 Eating Mindfully

Fall 2000 to Early 2001—age 24, 259 pounds and losing

August 15, 2000

When I got home this evening I had a fairly lengthy e-mail from Dad—telling Jeremiah and me about this woman he's started dating named Jackie.

My first reaction was that it was too soon. We haven't even buried Mom's ashes yet. I am trying to be adult about this, and in truth I don't feel like he's trying to replace Mom somehow. I know that he's been very lonely, but Jeremiah and I agree that Dad needs to have some consideration of how this will affect other people. It's only been very recently, after all, that we have begun to figure out our relationships with each other without Mom there as an interpreter or buffer, and we had barely begun to settle into our new roles—and now that's all blown out of the water.

My relationship with Dad has always been complicated, and in the past a lot of it has been angry. Since I've moved back to Maine, though, things were much better, and I felt like we finally had a real relationship. But talking to him tonight, all that was gone, and the old anger and impatience were back.

Jeremiah and I are both concerned at how quickly his life seems to be centering around this unknown woman, and what I guess I'm feeling right now is that I've already lost my mother, and now it feels like I'm losing my father that I was only just learning to appreciate having. I don't know if that makes sense, but that's how it feels. And then he was also going on about how Mom would have wanted him to move on with his life, and I don't disagree, but I don't think she meant for him to leave us behind.

Dad's dating upset me, but I knew I couldn't do much about it. Instead, I focused on what I could do: lose weight.

I started by paying more attention to my food choices, only to immediately encounter a stumbling block at work in the form of candy jars. Thea, who sat on one side, had a jar of peanut M&M's that seemed bottomless, since no sooner did it empty than she went to a nearby store to get more. The person who sat on my other side also had a candy jar, which didn't tempt me quite as much since the variety wasn't as appealing as the M&M's, but both proved hazardous.

"It's not fair," I complained to Shelly as we played rummy in my apartment. "It doesn't make it very easy to focus on losing weight."

She grinned. "Don't you remember *The Princess Bride?* We all know life isn't fair."

I laughed. "Good point."

"But how are you doing with the weight?"

"I haven't done much yet. Mostly I've been keeping a food journal for the past few days to see what I'm eating, and then Saturday I'm going to Dad's to get Mom's old hand weights." I sighed. "And that's annoying, too, because I had to remind him I didn't want Jackie to be there."

"Yeah. I still can't believe your dad started dating already." She put down all her cards. "I'm out."

We counted our points, and as I shuffled, I said, "I can't believe it, either. And he doesn't understand about me not wanting to meet her until after we bury Mom's ashes."

"That's coming right up, though, isn't it?"

I nodded and dealt another hand. "Just a couple more weeks. I know it normally would have happened already, but I do think it's important to have that finalized. Except then I won't have an excuse not to meet Jackie."

Listening to myself, I knew I sounded like a broken record, but I didn't know how else to handle the situation. None of my friends had dealt with parents remarrying, and the two of my uncles who had divorced didn't have any children. The idea of seeing Dad with someone other than Mom threw me off-balance, when I already teetered in a precarious position, with grief striking at odd times, hard enough that I still sometimes broke down in wrenching sobs.

My mind swarmed with all those thoughts when I drove to Casco Saturday morning. As soon as I arrived, Dad showed me the three-pound hand weights and two-pound ankle weights Mom had used. "Are these what you're looking for?"

"Yep." I realized I might graduate to heavier ones later, but for the moment, they looked good.

I put them in my backpack before sitting down at the table to talk. Dad started by asking, "So you're going to exercise more?"

"That's the plan. I want to start some strength training three days a week, and walk the other days."

He looked surprised. "You're going to do something every day?"

"I think I have to. If I skip a day, it's really easy to skip the next day, too, and then it just goes downhill." I remembered ruefully how often that had happened before.

"But you don't want to go to a gym." He made it half a statement, half a question.

I grinned. "A gym costs money."

He laughed sharply and clapped his hands. "Ha! That's my girl."

"Plus, I don't know any gyms on the bus line."

I didn't add how I simply couldn't face the idea of exercising in front of anyone. At my apartment, only my newly adopted cat, Salem, witnessed my activities. But she didn't care much about what I ate or did as long as I shared my tuna and turkey, provided cat food, and gave her plenty of attention.

"Well, good luck with it. I hope it works for you, since I don't think you want to do gastric bypass like Jackie did."

I managed not to grimace, both at the mention of Jackie and the idea of gastric bypass. I couldn't even contemplate that approach. "Definitely not. I'm not a fan of surgery in general, and isn't it also really expensive?"

"Oh, yeah. She saved up for years. But she doesn't regret it, since she lost over a hundred pounds."

I nodded politely and changed the subject. I suspected he wanted me to connect with Jackie over the weight issue, but I couldn't bring myself to talk more about her with the box of Mom's ashes a few feet away. Even now, I half-expected her to walk into the kitchen, maybe coming in from the garden, except without her ministrations, the garden had gone wild, already disappearing into weeds.

Back home in the evening, I considered how Dad talked non-stop about Jackie. He and Mom had been married for twenty-seven years, but it only took seven months for him to move on? And he didn't appreciate that even if he could find someone new to share his life, I would never have another mother.

Seemingly all by itself my hand opened a cupboard and reached for the chips. Only as I felt the cool bag and heard it crinkle did I pay attention to my actions.

I stopped and considered. I didn't particularly want a snack. I only wanted a distraction from thinking about Dad's relationship, and the chips were ready to oblige.

Part of me desperately wanted to eat them. Couldn't I wait until things quieted down before focusing on weight loss? Except when I thought about the past six years, I didn't know what "quiet" meant, between illness, marriage, birth, separation, and death.

If I kept using excuses, I would find something to keep me from losing weight forever. And it wasn't worth it. None of those things would be any different no matter how much or how little I ate.

With a strange sense of lightness, I put the chips back and deliberately closed the cupboard. I refused to let what other people did keep me from moving ahead with my own life any longer. A sense of victory lifted my heart, like I had cut free from something. Now I could finally focus on doing what I needed for me.

Fueled by my decision, I woke early the next morning to begin my new weight training routine. I didn't know many exercises, but even starting with leg lifts, arm curls, and a few attempted sit-ups counted as progress. To my surprise, I didn't mind it, although Salem looked confused as to why I got down on the floor and did such strange things.

I also studied my food journal and considered options. I could easily say I would only eat a certain number of calories, or cut out sweets, but did I really want to? Diets had always backfired for me.

Remembering that, I decided not to try another restrictive approach. I didn't want to categorically deny myself certain foods. I also realized I couldn't start something I would go "off" like a diet. I had to take an approach I could maintain forever, even if the idea of "forever" seemed overwhelming.

I started with modest changes. I stuck with juice and a big bowl of Cheerios for breakfast, and a turkey and soy cheese sandwich for lunch. Instead of pretzels or chips with the sandwich, I had veggies, then ended the meal with something sweet, a cookie or small brownie or chocolate graham cracker. For snacks I had fruit or pretzels instead of something sugary.

My evening meals changed the most, going from heavier foods to light fare like soup, usually from a can, or chef's salad, accompanied by fruit and chocolate soy milk. I might snack on a dessert later on, but nothing big. I also finished nibbling the chips in the cupboard, but I didn't buy more. For beverages, I started drinking more water, a *lot* more, and some herbal tea. At least I didn't have to overcome a soda addiction.

All went well except for the M&M's at work. I started each day intending to avoid them entirely, or have only a few. Then I'd get on the phone with a difficult customer support call and afterward grab a handful of candies to soothe myself. If work quieted down, the M&M's called me; eating gave me something to do. Or if someone else had them, the sound and sight of that person crunching through the sweet chocolate shell to the salty peanut made me want the same thing.

Once I started, I couldn't stop. Every time I went by Thea's desk—on the way to the door, the printer, the kitchen, and the bathroom—I'd take just a couple more. If I went the opposite direction, the candy jar on my other side tempted me. It all added up quickly. Drinking so much water didn't help, since I got up every hour either to pee or refill my bottle.

Despite those setbacks, I refused to beat myself up, since I hadn't put candy on a "forbidden" list. And even with the M&M's, when Shelly asked me how things were going the next week, I answered happily, "I've already lost two pounds!"

"That's great! Are you using the weights your dad gave you?"

"Yeah, and it's not that bad, especially if I watch something like *Buffy* while I'm doing it. So it's good."

"How much do you want to lose?"

I had given this a lot of thought. I had a vague idea of getting to 140, but it meant losing over a hundred pounds, an overwhelming concept. Instead, I told Shelly my short-term goal. "I want to start by losing twenty pounds by Christmas, and then go from there."

"Sounds reasonable. Good luck!"

I kept up with my walking and strength training and revised meals, but I soon realized I had more weaknesses than just the M&M's. Almost any food provided at work became a problem. One difficulty came with our tradition of celebrating everyone's birthday by getting cakes from Foley's, a local bakery. Their delicious confections of chocolate mousse and white chocolate mousse came artfully decorated with chocolate shavings and tasted simply divine.

When a birthday came up not long after I started losing weight, I tried to hold out at the gathering. I'd just had lunch. I didn't need a piece of cake. Then Thea passed the plates around, and I ended up holding one.

Maybe just a taste, I told myself. But, as with the M&M's, stopping proved much harder than starting. I ate the whole, wonderful slice.

I felt slightly guilty, but soon that gave way to physical problems: a queasy stomach and difficultly staying awake and focused. I wanted to take a nap.

"I'm not sure I should have had the cake." I yawned.

"No one said you had to," Thea said.

A revelation! Despite my heavy stomach, I straightened in my seat. Confronted by the cake, part of a celebration and looking delicious and creamy and rich, social conventions made me think I was supposed to eat it. In reality, though, no one would force me to, or care if I skipped it. It would simply mean more for everyone else. It helped when I realized Thea, also heavy, didn't let her size dictate what she ate.

Instead of worrying about what others thought, I could start paying attention to my body's needs. But I had a big problem.

I didn't know how to listen to my body.

11 Reclaiming My Body

Fall 2000 to Early 2001—age 24, 257 pounds and losing

September 8, 2000

I had an interesting evening. Jeremiah was having a movie night to show "The Matrix" on his new TV, and it was me, Patrice and Marcel, Dad—and Jackie. So we finally met her, but it was kind of odd. Actually, quite odd. She didn't talk much, and it was difficult to know what to say, and difficult to see Dad put his arm around her. I don't know. It's going to take a lot of getting used to.

I couldn't remember when I last had the urge to pay attention to my body on more than a superficial level. Maybe age ten or earlier, before the diets started, before I became convinced of my body's horrible, destructive nature as an all-consuming food machine. I tried for so long to pretend my physical self had nothing to do with me, it wasn't part of me at all, just something I got stuck with.

I knew I had to snap out of that. I needed to understand when I experienced true hunger or when I wanted to eat for other reasons like boredom, stress, loneliness, celebration, holidays, seeing someone else eat, and more. Unfortunately, I had no idea how. Then I found help from an unexpected source.

Exercise. It allowed me to focus on my body in a non-judgmental way, and after a short while I started noticing hunger signs. Not just growling stomach, but more subtle feelings of emptiness, losing the ability to focus, or noticing I became irritable when I needed to eat. I also simply felt better after I worked out or went for a walk, something I had never expected.

Curious, I asked Jeremiah, "Do you like exercising?"

"It depends on what it is. I can't stand using stationary bikes, but I love bike riding. And I like swimming and cross-country skiing and hiking, but not running. I also don't like group sports. Why do you ask?"

"I always assumed I hated all kinds of exercise—except maybe walking—because everyone in Dad's family has such a negative attitude about exercise. But now I wonder how much of that's really true, and how much I believed that because of being around them."

"I know what you mean. When I started on the cross-country ski team, I thought it would be horrible, but I really liked it."

After talking with Jeremiah, I started learning how to ignore habitual ideas about activity and hunger and food, focusing on my actual experience. I noticed exercise changed my hunger somehow, making it more genuine and easier to distinguish from other desires to eat.

This distinction became particularly clear one early November day when I left work stressed by some difficult customer support cases and still angry about a recent e-mail exchange with Dad, as I'd written in my journal.

> I sent an e-mail to Dad saying that I would prefer that this year the holidays be only for family, as last Christmas was really the last time we spent with Mom, and it's going to be difficult enough getting through it without Jackie being there.
>
> So now of course he comes back and says that he doesn't feel Jackie should be excluded from going to Patrice's on Christmas, since we're not enemies, and that no one else minds if she goes, and that his other option is to spend Christmas with Jackie's family. And really, he wrote, what would Mom think of this behavior? She would encourage us to live in the moment, not dwell on the past.
>
> So basically, he's trying to make me feel guilty for still grieving over Mom's death, even though he's been the one to say that different people grieve at different times. And, of course, it makes me look like a bitch for saying it at all, since everyone else has been so understanding and accommodating.
>
> I just don't know. I start crying whenever I even start to think about the holidays. Dad says that Jackie being there will make it easier for him, but I think it will just make it harder for me, because seeing her reminds me of what I've lost.
>
> But then it's really only Dad who's important, right? His feelings are the only valid ones.
>
> Maybe I'll just not do Christmas at Patrice's, but then Dad would accuse me of trying to be a martyr or making people feel sorry for me because I didn't get my way. I say this because that's the sort of thing he's said before. I'm tired of thinking about it, though.

Eventually we had compromised. Jackie would not be with us Christmas morning but would come by later in the afternoon. I continued simmering with lots of angst over the whole situation, though. Thinking about it vied for my attention with the work issues from the day, but I didn't want to deal with any of it.

Then, as soon as I stepped on the bus, I had a vision: chicken tenders and curly fries, both cooked to perfection, golden-brown and crispy and delicious and hot and fatty, with sweet and sour sauce and ketchup. My mouth watered. I thought how much I would enjoy it, how it would make me feel better, and after my long day and everything with Dad, I deserved it. I also knew I could easily get those foods from the Quality Shop, the convenience store right by my bus stop.

As the bus wound through the streets, though, I had time to think. Would getting take-out really make me feel better? By then, I knew eating too many rich foods, especially in the evening, often made my stomach protest. Emotionally it might help, but was that worth it? And I already had food at home. Should I spend money on a meal when I didn't need to?

When I reached my bus stop, I resolutely turned my back on the Quality Shop, despite its enticing aromas, and walked quickly home. I ate my normal supper and showered, all the while thinking about *why* I craved the chicken tenders and fries.

Then it hit me. Those were my comfort foods. I must be in need of comfort.

It made perfect sense and seemed obvious, but somehow I had never thought about it that way before. With the new perspective, I considered what else I might do. My video collection caught my eye, particularly one movie. I smiled and looked at Salem, who sat on the couch and purred, inviting me to pat her.

"What do you say to *Ghostbusters*?" I asked.

She just purred more, so I put in the movie. I alternated patting her silky black fur and doing some cross stitch, letting myself forget about my job and Dad's new relationship. The movie carried me back to a happier, simpler time of childhood, when Mom was still alive, and I laughed happily even though I knew all the punch lines.

It gave me what I needed: comfort viewing instead of comfort eating. I went to bed with an easy heart and a stomach that didn't complain.

By November 10, I had lost twelve pounds, and I could barely contain myself. It was working! I had more energy, my clothes fit a little better, and I didn't get out of breath quite so easily.

The panic therefore took me by surprise. It welled up in my chest, so strong I could hardly breathe. What was this? Why was I not happy? Why scared? I had to write it out to clarify for myself.

November 10, 2000

If I go through with this, which I have every intention of doing, I will at some point have to deal with the fact that I will be attractive.

That shouldn't be a scary thought, and yet somehow it is. Because in that case, if someone rejects me, I won't be able to have the comfortable, superior thought that it's because of my weight—it would be because of me.

And also, if I were attractive, I might actually get attention from men—which I would have no idea how to deal with. For years, I've been sort of subconsciously hoping for some man to like me, to validate me, despite my weight.

But something has changed, something to do with Mom's death and me getting on the scale this summer and realizing I had gained 20 pounds. I'm not doing this for my father's approval because, oddly and somewhat sadly, I no longer need it. But need it or not, when I get there, I might have that approval anyway, from him and others, and then what do I do with it? I have a while to figure it out, but still, it's a strange thought and one I wanted to jot down.

Although I didn't need Dad's approval, I soon found I still wanted it. By early December Jackie had as good as moved in with him, and I went to visit them just before Christmas.

Both of them wanted to know, "How are you doing with your weight loss?"

"I've lost seventeen pounds." I couldn't contain my pride. I hadn't lost so much weight consistently since those early days of Weight Watchers. But this felt incredibly different and better, knowing it came from *my* choice, *my* efforts.

Then Dad said, "That's rather slow."

I instantly deflated. I didn't know if he meant it to be critical, but that's how it came across. I tried not to show my crushing sorrow.

Before I could respond, Jackie said in a sharp, chiding tone, "Erik! You can do better than that." She looked back at me with a wide smile, "That's *awesome*, Erica. Congratulations! I can see it in your face. And it's smart to take your time. I would have done it that way if I could."

I struggled with a complex mix of emotions. I liked getting positive feedback, but why couldn't Dad be the one saying it? What should have been happy seemed suddenly fraught with tension, at least to me.

But I only said, "Thanks. And yeah, I'm definitely trying to go slow, since the weight's more likely to stay off."

Dad shrugged. "Well, good luck with it."

Jackie shook her head. "You should listen to your daughter. She's smart."

I escaped shortly after. While I appreciated Jackie's support, it only renewed my grief for Mom, who would have been my biggest cheerleader. Then came the guilt. Why had I let myself get so big, making Mom always worry about me? Why hadn't I lost the weight when she could have seen it? For a long time I sat alone in my living room, wracked and weeping.

In an odd way, grief for Mom and frustration about Dad's relationship and lack of encouragement helped me get through the holidays without loading up on food. It took so much energy for me not to cry or say what I really thought I didn't feel much like eating. By Christmas I had met my twenty-pound goal, but I didn't pause to celebrate. I still had a long way to go.

12 Ups and Downs

Early 2001 to Summer 2001—age 24–25, 235 pounds and losing

January 9, 2001

I wanted to write at least a bit today, since it's the first anniversary of Mom's death, and I can't believe, somehow, that it's already been a year. I was thinking about it last night, which would have been her 49th birthday, remembering how that night last year was one of the most difficult of my life.

Then this evening I was watching "Babylon 5", and it's at the point when Sheridan is on Z'ha'dum stuck between life and death. Delenn was watching one of his personal logs, and he said in it that his father always taught him to make something positive out of pain. It struck me because I had decided for myself, but partially forgotten, that the only way to really make sense of tragedies like Mom's death is to try to turn it into something positive, to grow from it.

And so today, I would like to think of what positive things I have gained in the past year. I have a deeper and more immediate appreciation of life, something I have especially noted recently with winter. A lot of people have complained about the snow and cold, but I am enjoying it. For the first time in years I helped make a snowman, and I found I do not mind shoveling, and I positively enjoy going for walks in the morning, seeing the world slowly emerge from black and white into color.

I have a greater appreciation of health, and therefore a greater determination to achieve it. I have realized the value of hard work and perseverance. I have understood better the value of laughter and the necessity of beauty.

In essence, I have learned to value everything more closely, and to appreciate what I have and can experience, knowing it is only temporary. I have grown up a lot in some ways in the past year, and while I would have been happier to wait a little longer to grow up, or to have Mom here to share in appreciating these things, I think the important thing is to recognize this as her legacy instead of sorrow, or at least in addition to the sorrow that is inevitable.

I still miss her at times more than I would think possible after a year, especially on nights like this when the mother moon shines full and bright, but at least I can choose to remember her as the vibrant, loving, graceful woman she was, not what she became in the hospital. It is with that memory and hope in my heart that I go tonight, seeking to create some positive growth out of this abiding pain.

Thinking of Mom only increased my determination to keep losing weight, but by the end of January, discouragement plagued me.

"I've still only lost a total of twenty pounds, not twenty-four or twenty-five like I'd hoped," I vented to Shelly on our way to have lunch at The Sedgley Place restaurant with my family.

"Has anything changed?" she asked.

"The only difference is I went to visit my college friend Steph. Mostly we ate at her house, and as a guest I felt like I should eat a fair amount of her mom's cooking, plus we also went out once." I sighed. "I gained four pounds!"

"Ouch."

"Yeah. I want to lose another twenty by my birthday, which is still doable as long as nothing else comes up and I can figure out how to deal with all the food at work. But I'll worry about that later. For today, I'm just going to enjoy the meal and company."

The irony did not occur to me until too late.

As we sat down at the restaurant, my stomach complained loudly. I had grown accustomed to eating between 11:30 and noon, and waiting until 12:30 meant I had gone beyond normal hunger to ravenous. I grabbed a roll as soon as I could, desperate for something to eat.

As I slathered butter on the bread, Patrice asked what now seemed a standard question, "How are you doing with losing weight?"

I winced. Maybe I didn't need quite as much butter. "Okay, but I don't think today will help."

"I know. Going out to eat is always hard, especially when the food is as good as it is here."

I nodded, but that didn't stop me from eating each course on the fixed price menu. Creamy vegetable soup. Garden salad. Chicken cordon bleu. My stomach grew increasingly full. I began to realize I couldn't eat this much in one sitting anymore. But I had already paid and wanted to get the full value of the meal. Maybe I should have taken some home. Even so, I couldn't resist dessert, nor did anyone else.

"I have a separate stomach for dessert," Dad told Marie solemnly.

She giggled, but when my brownie sundae arrived, I wished I really did have a different compartment for it. How else could I eat this huge piece of rich, fudgy, chocolaty goodness, with a generous topping of vanilla ice cream? I didn't feel the least bit hungry, but I knew the brownie would be delicious. I took a small bite then closed my eyes.

"Is it good?" Shelly asked, trying her cheesecake.

"It's awesome." Before I knew it, I took another bite, then another. Without quite realizing how, I finished it.

We all groaned as we stood. My waistband pressed uncomfortably against my expanded stomach. I shook my head, thinking of the overeating scene in Monty Python's *The Meaning of Life*.

"I'm not sure I could even eat a wafer thin mint."

Jeremiah caught the reference. "Better not to tempt it. It would be messy if you exploded."

"So nice to know your primary concern is the mess."

We waddled over to our coats, and I asked Dad and Jackie, "Will you be joining us to watch Chicken Run?"

"I don't think so," Dad said. "I need to emulate a snake after a big meal."

I grinned. "Nap time?"

"Yes."

Knowing they wouldn't be joining us at Jeremiah's relieved me. While Jackie had been supportive of me, seeing Dad with anyone other than Mom made me uncomfortable.

The rest of us went over for the movie, and by the time we arrived, I felt queasy. The fullness of my stomach made Jeremiah's question ironic.

"Did you guys bring chips?"

"Yep." I handed him the Doritos. "Although I don't think we need more food."

"It's part of the experience. We've got to have snacks for a movie."

I shook my head, especially when I saw how much we had: Doritos; Tostitos and salsa; crackers with three types of cheese; grapes; and carrots. "Do you really think we're going to eat all of this?"

He shrugged. "We'll eat what we can and have leftovers."

The movie started around 3:30, but at first the food distracted me. Incredulous, I realized it looked appealing. I munched on some Doritos and Tostitos. The saltiness helped settle my stomach. Then I went for the lighter and healthier grapes and carrots to balance out the earlier rich foods. I ate more of those than seemed possible.

Only after the movie ended did I pause to take stock of how I felt. I didn't like the results. I ran a real risk of throwing up. I didn't, but after a horrible night's sleep, the next morning I knew what a hangover would feel like. I had no energy, was queasy and dry-mouthed, and my brain didn't want to focus. I left work early and decided to never go that overboard again.

Luckily, as soon as I started taking more care with eating, the pounds dropped almost magically. At least, for a short time. Then I noticed a pattern.

February 24, 2001

I woke up this morning and was shocked to discover that I had somehow gained two pounds yesterday. I've kind of noticed before that at certain times of the month I can eat almost anything and lose weight, and other times even being really careful it's a struggle just to maintain. It seems to be tied to my cycle, and now I think I'm in the latter part, which is about a month since I visited Steph and gained four pounds, so there is a pattern. Hopefully in another week or so I'll lose again.

The pattern held, and by March 4, I smiled in delight at the numbers on the scale. "I've lost thirty pounds!" I told Thea as soon as I arrived at work, needing to share my excitement.

"Congratulations! It's definitely showing. How does it feel?"

"Pretty incredible." I couldn't stop smiling. "I mean, I still have a long ways to go, but I'm a quarter of the way, and I've never lost this much weight all at once. I'm excited to buy new clothes, and I'm also doing better with sweets, so I'm going to try an experiment."

When I pulled out my sandwich bag with a few peanut M&M's, she looked confused. "I already have M&M's."

"I know, but this way I can keep track of how many I'm eating. I'm not telling myself I can't have any, but this is it for the day."

She nodded slowly. "Okay, I can see that."

As I went through the day, every time I felt tempted by the candy jar, I took one or two of my M&M's. I even had a few left by the time I went home, making me feel good. My only regret, as always, came from not being able to share my success with Mom.

Sorrow hit even harder on March 20 when I read Dad's e-mail. After enthusing about a visit to the Flower Show, he dropped a bombshell. "Oh, and I have some news. I proposed to Jackie today, and she accepted! We're both very excited about it."

I stared at the screen. I didn't have the faintest idea how to respond. At least he hadn't told me over the phone; this way I could get my emotions under control. Easier said than done.

March 20, 2001

What the hell do I say? Congratulations? Is there a reason he proposed on the first day of spring? Will I have to explain that I won't refer to her as my stepmother? I'm so confused! That's my predominant emotion, that and some frustration—I didn't need any more stress in my life right now, really I didn't.

Trial by fire, I thought. At any earlier time in my life, I would have turned to food, but not this time. Instead, the emotional energy gave me fuel for another life change I'd had in mind ever since my landlords sold my building and I'd had to switch units so the new owners could live in my apartment.

I decided to buy my own place.

"Why is that related to your dad getting remarried?" Shelly asked when I told her.

"Because it made me realize that house will never be home again, especially since Jackie is redecorating and making my old room into her 'nest', according to Dad. I simply want something more permanent than I have, where I'm not dangling at the whim of the landlord. Plus, since Dad asked me to get everything of mine out of the house, I could use the extra space."

"Makes sense. Good luck with it."

The luck came through. I saw a realtor on a Tuesday, and after a whirlwind week had my offer accepted on a condo the following Sunday. On May 9, I moved a mile away from the apartment. Settling in took some time, but Salem and I liked our new home. Even better, I discovered I could still walk to Evergreen Cemetery and visit Gov. Baxter's headstone. Being reminded of Baxter State Park helped me focus, for weight loss and to be able to climb Katahdin again.

Through it all I tried to be mindful of my eating, but I didn't know what to expect on May 28 when I stepped on the scale. Then I saw the numbers—219!

I breathed a relieved sigh, and when Patrice called to wish me happy birthday, I shared the good news. "I met my goal. I've lost forty pounds!"

"Congratulations!" I smiled at the pride in her voice. "That's so wonderful!"

"Yes, it is. Especially since it means I now have less than a hundred pounds to go." I'd reached a major milestone.

Only later did I realize I didn't share some of the emotions of my family and friends.

July 11, 2001

The odd thing is that while other people may be proud of me for losing weight, I'm not exactly proud of it myself. It's not a matter of thought or pride for me—it's simply something I'm doing, period. It would be like being proud of myself for brushing my hair or my teeth; it doesn't make sense to me. Of course, I'm not sure that would make sense to anyone else, but there you have it.

It put me in a thoughtful mood and made me somehow even more determined to go hiking when I went to Baxter State Park on July 21. I decided once more to attempt Katahdin Stream Falls, this time with my friend Steph since Shelly couldn't join us.

Steph and I hiked at a moderate rate, stopping occasionally for water, but now it seemed like I floated along. I didn't struggle to breathe! I didn't turn bright red! I could hear the sounds of the forest and falls, not just my furiously pumping blood. Not once did I stop for a break, other than a nature call. Not once did I have to chide myself out of despair in order to keep moving. I couldn't have been happier.

We paused when we arrived at the bottom of the falls, and Steph said, "Wow. That's gorgeous."

"Yes, it is." I had never appreciated it more.

We proceeded to the top, and I even managed the steep scramble up the huge boulders with relative ease. After we took in the scene, Steph suggested, "We should swap places and get each other's pictures down there and up here."

"Sounds good."

As I headed down to the low viewpoint, it hit me. Without even thinking about it, I had agreed to climb up a small portion of the trail twice, something I never would have done before.

It made the way down much more pleasant. Once back at the campsite, I told Dad, "The hike was great! And so much easier this time."

He nodded. "You look fine, not really tired."

"I'm not." My legs didn't feel sore, and my shirt was only damp, not soaked, with sweat.

"So what made you decide to lose weight?"

I'd thought a lot about how I might answer that question, but I hadn't expected it to come from Dad. "When I saw what Mom went through with cancer, I realized if I ever have to experience that, I wanted to know what it's like to be healthy first. I couldn't keep putting it off, because I don't know how long I have, given how young she died."

I choked up and had to stop. Dad looked thoughtful as he crossed his arms over his large stomach. "I thought it might be to climb Katahdin again."

"That's part of it," I admitted. "But it was really everything together."

I couldn't bring myself to say I had also given up seeking his or other people's approval. I was simply happy to have that much of a conversation, which showed renewed progress in our relationship.

We settled in for the afternoon, and I already had my goal for next year: to get to Chimney Pond without it nearly killing me.

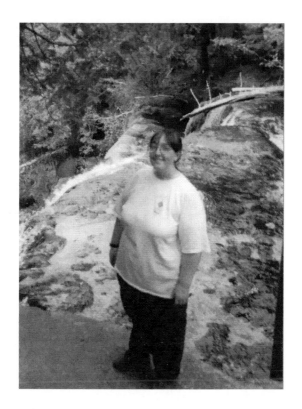

July 2001, Erica at the top of Katahdin Stream Falls

13 Baggage Check

Late 2001 to early 2002—age 25, 210 pounds and losing

July 31, 2001

I've been reflecting on my weight loss, now that I'm down forty-nine pounds, and I've noticed I don't obsess about my size anymore. I don't let my weight get me depressed, I don't think about how hideous I am, or what other people must think when they look at me—because thinking about it only ever got me depressed and angry and disinclined to do much beyond sulk and complain, which is hardly productive. Instead, I am simply doing it, with defeat not even a possibility in my mind.

On the morning of August 4, 2001, I stood with Shelly in the lobby of my church. Dad and Jackie would be getting married in less than an hour. I couldn't live in denial much longer.

"How are you holding up?" Shelly asked.

I shrugged. "I'm trying not to think about it much. I mean, I know Mom would have wanted Dad to be happy, but it's so fast. I'm also confused about why Mémère and Pépère are here." I nodded to where Mom's parents sat in the sanctuary. "They almost boycotted Mom and Dad's wedding, and they've never been overly fond of Dad."

Shelly gave me a hug. "Hard to say, but hang in there." Then she smiled. "And hey, at least you have a fancy new size eighteen dress to wear!"

"True." I smiled despite myself. I hadn't fit in a size eighteen for a long time.

After a seeming eternity of waiting, the ceremony began, and thankfully it went quickly. I knew lunch wouldn't start immediately, between photos and setting up the buffet, which left me plenty of time to visit guests.

I found myself standing next to Mémère and Pépère. Even in the best of times, I rarely knew what to say to them. We had never been very close, especially since Mémère didn't approve of my large size. My weight loss, though, gave her something to talk about.

"Oh, Erica!" Mémère gave me a big smile when she saw me. "You look so good. I can really see that you've lost a lot of weight."

"Thank you." I tried to hide my mix of emotions: pleasure at the compliment, annoyance about her consistent focus on my weight, and continued incredulity at her presence.

"I'm so proud of you, and it's not only your weight. You've changed. You're much friendlier than you used to be."

"You think so?"

"Oh, yes." Her tone left no possibility of doubt.

I didn't disagree, but having Mémère, who rarely saw me, be the first person to comment on it intrigued me. After mulling it over, I wrote in my journal:

> *August 10, 2011*
>
> *Since Mom died, my personality has changed, though Mémère is the first to comment on it. I realized all this crap I was carrying around, angst and depression and shame, things that made me very shy and withdrawn because I believed no one would want to talk to me, or touch me, or take any pleasure in my company because of my weight, was just that—crap. If people don't want to talk to me or be around me, odds are that's their problem as much as mine, and they're probably not the sort of people I want to be around anyway.*
>
> *And so I started to be more outgoing. Nothing like Jeremiah, mind you, but more willing to talk to people I don't know, with a feeling that I can relate more to them now, as if I'm more rooted in ordinary life because of Mom's death. The people I work with, especially Thea, have also helped, showing me that just because you're overweight doesn't mean you have to let other people treat you badly.*
>
> *And I'm not going to haul around all the old wounds of people making fun of me, and my feeling grotesque any longer, because I have enough weight as it is—that only overburdens me, holding me down from moving on with my life.*

After thinking it through, I felt lighter. Not worrying about the opinions of other people made me so much happier and increased my confidence.

My happiness went up another level not long after when I received an invitation to a wedding I couldn't wait to attend.

"I'm going to Ireland!" I told Shelly.

"What? When?"

"My Irish friend David, the one I met during my study abroad in England, is getting married at the end of February. I figured I'll never get invited to a wedding in Ireland again, so I'm doing a whirlwind weekend trip. And it's great because our friend Nina, who was in England with me and David, will be coming from Belgium for the wedding, so we'll get to hang out again."

"That's awesome! And I'm only moderately jealous of you getting to go to Ireland."

Others responded in similar ways. On Thanksgiving, my aunt Annette even asked, "Are you sure you don't need a nurse to go with you, maybe smuggled in your luggage?"

I grinned. "I'm sure."

"Too bad." Then her eyes lit up with excitement again. "But you're going to need a new dress!"

I barely swallowed my piece of pie before laughing. "I guess so. I hadn't really thought about it, but I do have to say it's pretty awesome to buy new, smaller clothes these days."

She smiled. "I can imagine. It's always one of the things I like when I'm able to lose a little weight. You should check out Chadwicks online. They have a lot of good options."

"Thanks. It'll be exciting to get a more normal-sized dress."

Jeremiah overheard us and commented, "I don't see why the clothes thing is such a big deal."

Since I knew he'd also been losing a little weight, I asked, "So what's your motivation?"

"I know for every pound I lose, I'm that much closer to having sex." I laughed. "You think I'm joking?"

"No. That's why it's funny."

Despite my laughter, a wave of uncertainty swept through me. Although I didn't share Jeremiah's goal of losing weight to have sex, I knew with each lost pound I became more conventionally attractive. Eventually men might notice me! Including those like Chris, who tried to take advantage of me when I had been hopelessly overweight.

No one had ever discussed this aspect of weight loss with me. I wondered why. In some ways becoming normal looking, and even attractive, represented a more drastic change than the weight itself.

How do you learn to respond if someone hits on you, whether or not you're interested? How do you start to see yourself as beautiful on the outside as well as inside, when your whole life has been labeled the opposite? How do you handle compliments? How do you accept and claim your new body? And how do you deal with the fear of how other people might treat you?

I took a deep breath. I didn't have to worry about it yet. I still had another sixty or seventy pounds before I entered dangerous territory. Instead, I wanted to appreciate how far I'd come and celebrate by buying a new dress for my friend's wedding.

With that in mind, I took Annette's advice and looked at Chadwicks. com. Then I realized I didn't know my size. For years, my method of finding the right sized clothes involved trying things on until something fit, not an option for purchasing online.

I went into my bedroom and stripped down to my underwear to accurately measure my waist, hips, and bust. As I jotted down the numbers, it hit me. Here I stood, nearly naked, focusing on my body, and not freaking out. That had never happened before.

Previously I'd been uneasy when undressed, afraid of what I might see if I accidentally glanced down, knowing how grotesque my body had become. While I still had a long ways to go, a new and unexpected feeling swept through me: appreciation of and fondness for this body. Even more, acceptance of it as mine, not something I wanted to disinherit.

I put on a T-shirt and looked in the mirror. Instead of focusing on all my flaws, I noticed the good things. I could see my collarbones and wrist bones. When I flexed my fingers, tendons danced visibly beneath my skin. My double chin, while not completely gone, had receded notably. For the first time I could imagine reclaiming some of the inherent grace and beauty with which I'd been born.

It made me happy and excited again. I realized I could start taking compliments by first acknowledging my worth to myself.

I loved the idea, but it didn't help with buying a dress, especially when I realized I wouldn't be able to get one in the right size even with the measurements. I planned to lose more weight between now and the wedding, and the dress problem would grow as I shrank. Then I remembered how Patrice and I used to make some of my clothes. I gave her a call.

"I have a favor to ask. I want to order a dress for David's wedding, but I'll probably have to guess at the size. If it's a little too big, can you help me take it in before I leave?"

"Of course. And it's so wonderful that you'll get to go, and you're still losing weight."

"Yeah, it really is." I smiled, this time feeling only the pleasure without the panic.

By mid-February 2002 I had lost over eighty-five pounds, down to about 170, and I decided I wouldn't lose much more before the wedding. I ordered a dress, then brought it—and my new body—to Patrice's.

As she tucked and pinned, she asked, "So will you be sticking to your diet while you're there? I mean, I know you're not doing a regular diet, but will you still try to eat healthily?"

"To some extent."

"Do you mind me asking what you eat these days?"

"Not at all. I have Cheerios for breakfast, with chocolate soy milk on the side. I have half a sandwich, some veggies, and most days a fruit with lunch, and snacks of pretzels or fruit. And dinner is usually salad or soup or another vegetable dish, some type of protein, and maybe another fruit. That's generally about it. I might have a piece of chocolate in the evening, but I try not to snack a lot then."

"I can see why you're losing!"

"Well, the funny thing is, my eating isn't much about the weight anymore. I simply feel better if I eat healthy foods—better physically, I mean—but I feel lousy if I eat too much sugar or fat or fried stuff. So it makes sense to eat those foods in moderation."

"Good for you. I have to say I've never had that problem when I eat lots of sugar."

"I didn't used to, but last Halloween I didn't even want the candy I bought for trick-or-treaters. What I had at work was plenty." I didn't tell her I snuck some candy back to the kitchen at work, having taken too much and getting an upset stomach from the little I ate. "I'm also more willing to try new foods when I travel for work, like seafood and fancy dishes, which will help."

"Definitely." Patrice made a couple more adjustments. "Take a look and let me know what you think, but be careful not to move too much or you'll hit some pins."

I went into her bedroom and looked in the mirror. I could hardly believe the reflection. Could this be me? At Christmas, Mom's family had said how much I looked like her, and now I started seeing it, too. I blinked back tears.

"It's perfect, Patrice. Thank you."

I flew to Ireland the night of February 26, and I couldn't believe how easy travel seemed. I fit in the seat without overflowing the arm rests, and I could walk down the narrow aisles and use the tiny bathroom without worrying I might get stuck. Managing my luggage didn't exhaust me, and when the person in front of me leaned the seat back I didn't feel completely trapped.

It all put me in a very good mood, despite being tired, when I arrived in Cork on February 27. David and Nina met me at the airport, and they looked almost exactly the same even after four and a half years. Nina, also heavyset, had shrunk a little, but neither had changed drastically. They had a different reaction, though, upon seeing me.

"Oh my God!" Nina stared at me, her lovely gray eyes wide. "I almost didn't recognize you! You're so thin!" She turned to David. "Isn't she skinny?"

David froze a moment at being put on the spot, but he rallied. "You look grand."

"Thanks." We exchanged hugs, and I smiled widely, realizing how much I'd missed them. "It's great to see you guys."

I had a wonderful weekend. I loved hearing all the Irish accents, going to Timoleague and Skibbereen, staying in Lettercolum House, and trying the different foods. I worried, though, about how much I ate at the wedding feast.

Nina and I sat at a round table with the bride and groom and a couple of their friends, and at the start, the odor of warm rolls enticed me. I treated myself to one before our excellent meal began. For an appetizer I had a tartlet made with tomatoes, tangy and creamy goat cheese, and herbs, with a garden salad on the side. My main course, a tender and succulent rack of lamb, came surrounded by roast potatoes, carrots, green beans, and cabbage. I left the carrots, not liking them cooked, but everything else tasted wonderful.

By then very full, if not quite to bursting, I appreciated my outfit's lack of a waistband. Then another dish appeared: pears in red wine sauce with vanilla ice cream.

"Don't you have wedding cake in Ireland?" I asked David.

"We do, after the dessert. And be glad Fiona and I are breaking with tradition on that."

"Why?"

"Irish weddings have fruit cake, and it's just *awful*. It's hard as a rock and no one eats it."

I laughed as he made a face. "So what kind of cake are you having instead?"

"Chocolate."

I debated internally. The pear and ice cream looked good. I also wanted the cake. I didn't need either, let alone both, but for a once-in-a-lifetime event, I could splurge, as long as I didn't make myself sick.

I compromised by having a little taste of the excellent pear and ice cream. Then we had a break for toasts and conversation before the cake came, topped with a sparkler in the shape of a heart. I enjoyed a small but delicious piece.

In the end, I knew I had eaten too much but decided not to worry about it. Still, when I flew home the next day, getting back to my normal habits came as a relief. I hadn't realized until then how much I missed my usual exercise and food, and I wanted to get back on track to make my next goal: bring my total weight loss to one hundred pounds by my birthday.

14 Becoming My Own Heroine

Spring and Summer 2002—age 25–26, 164 pounds and losing

March 2002

I took my measurements to help determine what sizes I should look for at J.C. Penny, and it's really exciting not to have to look at plus sizes anymore! It's a very strange concept for me, since I've never been able to shop in the regular part of the store until recently, and I'm going to have to be careful not to go too crazy.

The weight kept dropping, and by mid-April I had lost ninety-five pounds. My pleasure and excitement at continuing to meet my goals increased when I discovered all the things I could do with my changing body.

Crossing my legs offered a whole new experience, and fitting through narrower spaces gave me great joy. I could squat down to Marie's six-year-old level, then rise without using my hands. Shirts with buttons didn't run the risk of popping or gaping open. I could walk short distances in a skirt without my thighs rubbing each other raw.

To most people, these might be small things, but to me, they marked significant triumphs. Even better, I had entered a positive feedback loop. The more I lost, the better I felt and the more determined to reach my goals.

But I didn't think about how others perceived me. I assumed, as I had in my teen years, that if anyone noticed me at all, it would be in a negative way. Until the compliments started.

One of my coworkers in customer support told me, "I'm so impressed with your weight loss. You're my inspiration." Seeing my expression, she said, "I'm serious. I really mean that."

"Thank you." What she said honored and touched me, knowing she also wanted to slim down.

Then a lovely e-mail came from one of our tech writers: "I just wanted to send you a note to say that I am incredibly impressed at how WONDERFUL you look—I don't know what you're doing or how you're managing to do it, but you look great! I have infinite admiration for what you've accomplished—keep up the good work—you are amazing!!!" It gave me a warm, fuzzy feeling all afternoon.

A funnier moment came when one of the testers said, "You don't have a butt anymore!" Seeing my expression, she added quickly, "I mean that in a good way."

Not long after, Thea also said, "You look really good." I had to laugh. "What?"

"It's funny because everyone seems to be coming out of the woodwork with compliments. It's cool, but I don't know why it's happening all of a sudden."

"Didn't you just get some new clothes?"

"Yeah." I'd recently spent a whole evening making room by weeding out my closet and having fun making up four bags of clothes for Goodwill.

"That's probably part of it. Plus, how often do you meet someone who's lost so much weight on their own?"

I could see her point, but even so, the comments felt strange. Never had I thought I would inspire or impress people in any physical sense. At a stretch, maybe with my academics or writing. But weight loss? It seemed surreal.

That feeling increased when one of my co-workers asked, "Do you mind me asking what you're doing to lose weight?"

What a contrast to all those years of negative conversations about food and weight. I couldn't help wondering, though, if she hoped for an easy answer, some quick fix, the same thing I used to dream about.

"Nothing too extreme," I said. "Mostly paying more attention to what I eat and adding some exercise."

"If you have time, could you send me an e-mail with what you're eating? It might give me some ideas."

I nearly laughed at someone asking me for food advice. "I'd be happy to."

I soon noticed another change: I had somehow become social. In addition to my usual solitary pursuits like writing, reading, and cross-stitch, I often visited family and friends, started doing more with church (particularly with lay-led worship), had joined a book group, and generally became more active.

Dad even commented in an e-mail, "Your social calendar seems to have grown in proportion to your weight loss." I couldn't argue, and I found I liked it.

My self-confidence rose by mid-May, when I had lost ninety-nine pounds. Then I hit a plateau. After two weeks, when I realized I would miss my one hundred pound goal, I panicked. I didn't think I had changed anything. Not sure what else to do, I kept a food journal again to see what I might have missed.

As I looked over my notes, I realized social events still tripped me up. Seeing how much others ate gave me the sense I should eat the same way, even though I didn't need much food. Eating anywhere close to what others usually did was too much.

Once I started paying attention to that and didn't eat simply to keep up with others, my weight loss resumed. My scale read 159—my one hundred pound goal—right after my birthday.

I breathed a deep sigh of relief. I had another twenty or thirty pounds to go, and I didn't want to get stuck, knowing I still had the hike up Katahdin ahead of me. For this year, though, my goal remained getting to Chimney Pond without feeling horrible.

When we headed to Baxter State Park on July 13, I asked Shelly, "Are you up for going to Chimney Pond again?"

"Absolutely! Do you think you'd want to go higher?"

"Let's play it by ear and see how we're doing when we get there." My confidence didn't extend quite that far, but if I did take a chance on going farther, I'd be able to scatter some of Mom's ashes, safe in the small film canister Dad had given me.

Jeremiah and our two college friends, Janice and Dan, also planned on hiking, but Shelly and I finished getting ready to leave first. We waited a minute before I said, "Why don't we just start. I'm sure they'll catch up."

She agreed, and we started on the trail. When Jeremiah, Janice, and Dan didn't appear, I took stock of my physical condition, an incredible difference from previous years. I barely noticed the steeper section, too caught up in conversation and hearing about Shelly's online dating attempts. I did slow down, and occasionally Shelly drew ahead of me, but in general we kept our initial pace. Not once did I have to force myself to start up an incline, I didn't gasp for breath or feel creeping despair. I couldn't have been happier.

At Chimney Pond, I stopped, stunned. "We're here already?" I glanced at my watch. "We did a little over three miles in two hours?"

Shelly laughed and gave me a hug. "Congratulations!"

Pleased but incredulous, I followed her to the edge of the pond. It seemed even more beautiful than I remembered because this time I could look at it with ease, standing strong and capable, not staggering in after four hours with the last of my strength. I took in the glittering water and gorgeous landscape, tears in my eyes.

A few minutes later, Jeremiah, Janice, and Dan arrived, and they quickly joined us in taking off backpacks and having a snack on the rocks by the water.

"Better than last time?" Jeremiah asked as he munched on trail mix.

"Infinitely," I said with feeling, pulling out my own trail mix and grapes.

"Do you want to go on?" Shelly asked.

"I don't know. What is everyone else doing?"

"We want to try Cathedral Trail," Jeremiah said.

I hesitated. I remembered Dad's story of becoming dehydrated while on that trail and hallucinating about being in hell. It didn't motivate me.

"We could always turn back if it's too much," Shelly pointed out.

I capitulated. I felt good; I could at least start it. "Okay, I'll give it a try."

We left Chimney Pond about 10:45, and I began at what seemed like the same pace as before. My confidence flagged when, in a matter of minutes, Jeremiah, Dan and Shelly pulled far ahead.

Discouraged, I pressed on. I couldn't give up this soon. Then Janice and I reached the bottom of an incline that made me realize why this route was a half-mile shorter than the other option, the Saddle Trail. The path rose steeply, composed almost entirely of rocks of all shapes and sizes, everything from boulders to loose shale.

Janice said, "I hate to say this, but once you go up that, I don't think you can turn back."

I stared at the intimidating path, heart sinking. I imagined coming down. It would be downright treacherous. I swallowed bitterly. We had already agreed that none of us would hike alone, so turning back now would force Janice to return with me. We also didn't have any way to tell the others about a change of plan. I had little choice.

Resigned, I settled my backpack as comfortably as I could and said, "Let's go."

Clambering over the rocks started off fun. It got old fast, though. I envied Janice's long legs, wishing mine had a few extra inches. By the time we caught up with the others where they waited for us, I knew this had been a mistake.

"How are you doing?" Shelly asked.

"Not great. This isn't really what I expected."

"Do you want to go back?"

I tried not to sound bitter. "I think it's too dangerous for me to try getting down the trail, so I have to keep going, at least to the cut-over to the Saddle Trail."

Shelly didn't argue. Instead, she offered, "Let us know if we can help."

"Okay."

And everyone did help, a lot. They sometimes carried my backpack, and other times gave me a hand or boost to get past spots I simply couldn't do alone. I appreciated it even as I hated feeling like a burden. Not having my backpack on hand also backfired, since it meant I didn't drink enough water and quickly became dehydrated.

My world narrowed to my immediate obstacles. I no longer enjoyed the rocks, or noticed their beauty. I simply had to move past them so I could turn around and get down. Each time I came to a daunting set of boulders, I stopped to consider my options. Should I go left, right, straight? Did the footing look stable?

I moved carefully, testing each step before committing, bracing and pulling with my hands, palms slightly raw from the rough stone. My muscles ached and joints protested. For the first time in a couple of years I felt despair, and anger at myself for agreeing to this, and disappointment with my body's limitations. I came close to hating the hike.

That added to my teetering emotional state. I couldn't stop thinking about Mom, and how I wanted climbing to be a joyful experience. Had I stopped at Chimney Pond, it would have been, but now I couldn't even appreciate the views.

In a rare moment alone, I stopped to collect myself. I sat on a boulder and faced the way we came. As my breathing slowed and the utter quiet and peace settled over me, I finally registered the spectacular scenery. The rock field held rugged charm, the geometric jumble a whole array of gray and tan and ochre shades against the clear sky. Very few plants survived this high up, but lichen formed intricate patterns on some rocks. The mountain looked stripped down, clean, and in every way elemental.

I decided to take some pictures, but after one shot my camera ran out of film. I reached into my bag for a new roll, but the canister I grabbed didn't have film. It held Mom's ashes.

I broke down. Sobs wracked me, though I barely had enough moisture for tears. I wept not only from lack of ability but a sense of abandonment and isolation. Everyone else forged on happily ahead, without the burden of grief and angst towards their body I carried. Even Jeremiah wouldn't feel it as much, having climbed Katahdin with Mom multiple times and having scattered his own set of ashes the year before.

Sick with dejection, I snuffled my way through a handful of tissues until gaining composure. How could I keep going? I was beat. I no longer wanted to see or talk to anyone; I preferred being alone with my grief. Yet what choice did I have? I simply had to find the strength.

I put the ashes safely away, changed my film, picked myself up, and headed on. I found Jeremiah waiting a couple of boulders up. "Are you okay?"

"Not really." I tried not to sound bitter or weepy, but I don't know how well I managed. "But there's not much I can do about it." I could see he wanted to offer some encouragement but didn't know what. "I just need to get to the cut-off to Saddle Trail. There's no way I'm making it to the top."

"Well, hopefully that won't be long."

I knew it couldn't be far, but even so I didn't arrive until 2 p.m., struggling every step of the way to keep my battered and bruised self going.

I must have looked on the verge of collapse because Shelly asked, "Do you want me to stay with you?"

I knew everyone else planned to go to the top, and while I appreciated the offer, I didn't want to deny her that chance as I had so many other years. Plus, I would have a little time alone.

"No, I'll be fine. I'm sure you'll catch up soon."

Despite knowing how fast they went, I couldn't believe Shelly and Dan made it to the top then caught up with me almost as soon as I reached the Saddle Trail. They proceeded down, easily outpacing me, and looking hardly the worse for wear. I tried, again, not to be bitter.

Jeremiah and Janice stayed with me most of the way, sometimes carrying my backpack. Talking with them about recent episodes of *Buffy the Vampire Slayer* and *Angel* finally lifted my spirits, as did gravity, helping not hindering. Dan took over companion duties for the last mile, having come back up the trail after shooting ahead and checking in. Discussing fantasy and sci-fi books with him kept me going until I limped into the ranger's station at 8:30, eleven hours after starting.

Dan left me at my lean-to. "I'll let everyone else know you're here. Join us when you can."

"Thanks."

Extreme exhaustion meant cleaning up took half an hour and almost an entire container of Wet Wipes; I had accumulated an astonishing amount of dirt. But the process helped, as did wearing sandals and clean clothes. I hobbled to the other lean-to.

"Woo hoo!" Jackie said with a big smile. "You made it!" Everyone else smiled and clapped.

"Barely," I said, flustered by her enthusiasm. "And with a lot of help."

"Still, congratulations!"

Confused, I muttered, "Thanks."

Nothing except exhaustion really registered. I forced myself to eat a little—an apple, Fritos, some bacon, bell pepper, and cookies—while the others had the more usual fare of BLTs, chips, cookies, and hot chocolate. I had barely enough energy to brush and braid my hair before crashing.

The next morning I woke early, stiff and sore, but not in as bad shape as my first climb to Chimney Pond. When I returned from a slow trip to the outhouse, Shelly said, "I didn't get a chance to tell you yesterday, but I'm so proud of you for doing the climb, and so is everyone else."

"Thanks. But I wouldn't have done if it I'd known what it would be like, or if I'd had a choice."

"I know, but it's still an accomplishment."

It didn't feel like one to me, but I didn't argue.

I arrived home by early afternoon and unpacked in slow motion before showering. The hot water washed over me deliciously, warming my face and carrying the lingering dirt down the drain. Relaxed, I took stock. I could walk but had a spectacular set of bruises, including on my toenails. I worried I would lose them. I had also gained back a few pounds at Baxter, my overeating trumping all the exercise.

I checked e-mail and an unexpected note from Dad cheered me. "Jackie and I are awed by what you did. We didn't think you'd go further than Chimney Pond."

Did I deserve their praise? How could I consider it an accomplishment when it brought so much anguish, throwing me back to my younger years of hating my body?

And yet—I had gone far, coming close to Baxter Peak. That meant I *could* do it, and now I could prepare more effectively. I began feeling better, my confidence slowly inching back up.

Another boost came when reading *The Armless Maiden—and Other Tales of Childhood's Survivors*, edited by Terri Windling. Her introduction touched me deeply, as I wrote in my journal.

> *Windling pointed out the value of such stories as 'The Armless Maiden', saying how they remind us that we can find our way out of the woods through our own persistence and strength, that we can transform ourselves. This rang very true for me because for too long I allowed myself to feel victimized. But now I am finally acting, on a path out of the darkest woods and on the road to freedom.*

Thinking about it exhilarated me. At first I didn't know why. Then I realized. I had stopped waiting for anyone else to save me. I had taken action and wasn't far from meeting goals that once seemed impossible.

I had become my own heroine.

15 Unexpected Gifts

Summer 2002 to December 2002—age 26, 154 pounds and losing

July 27, 2002

I used to dread doing anything that would attract attention, positive or negative, because I was sure that anyone who actually focused on me would be disgusted because of my weight. But I'm not really worrying about that anymore. I'm no longer disgusted by myself, so at this point I tend to think that if anyone else reacts that way to me, it's because they have their own issues to deal with. So I smile and say hello when I'm out walking, and I'll actually ask for help or information at stores, etc. I find it's actually rather pleasant to be able to go through life without worrying so much about what people think of my appearance, and I think it's freed up a lot of energy for other things.

After the trip to Baxter State Park, I wanted to lose a little more weight, and I knew I could. But I did have a problem.

I had grown sick and tired of the whole process.

I wanted to be finished. I had this strange sense that my life had been put on hold until I reached my goal, but after two years, I didn't want to wait any longer.

I made a radical decision in the hope of speeding up the weight loss. I cut out sugar. No more peanut M&M's or cake or cookies. I didn't know how well it would work, remembering my earlier craving for sweets, but this time was different. I could think about how good something would taste, and then I remembered my goals and wasn't tempted. I had become deaf to that siren call.

A virtuous glow filled me, but it soon faded when I found I now ate so little that food became an obsession. In quiet times at work, I occasionally fantasized about eating—usually healthier options like apples and cucumbers instead of sweets—counting down the minutes until I could eat again.

Drinking tea and chewing gum helped distract me, but not always. Only if I couldn't concentrate did I succumb and have a snack. Being so hungry sometimes didn't feel quite right, but I kept losing, and that had become my overriding goal. As long as the hunger wasn't constant, I told myself not to worry.

Until I hit another plateau.

This one made me panic more than the first. After all, how much else could I do? Then I had another revelation when I considered my habits. I had been eating too much healthy food.

What a bizarre concept! It took me a while to accept it as reality. After all, I had never heard anyone talk about the possibility of too many apples, carrots, tomatoes, salads, etc. But in reality, I needed very little. When I counted my average calories out of curiosity, they came in around 1,000.

By myself, I could manage eating so little. Around other people, even when I wasn't hungry I felt like I *should* eat more, but this time not in an effort to keep up with them. Given how much they took in, it simply seemed logical to eat the same amount in order to keep my body going, even if my body didn't agree.

When I stopped comparing myself to others and listened to my body, I started losing again. What a relief! By mid-October I had lost 115 pounds, getting down to 144. This triggered another round of compliments.

A co-worker told me, "I passed you the other day when you were standing at the bus stop, but I almost didn't recognize you because there's so much less of you!"

I had to grin. "Thanks."

A woman whose house I passed while walking stopped me one morning to ask, "Are you the one I saw walking all winter?"

"Yes."

"Well, you look great. Keep it up!"

I moved on with a spring in my step.

Then the holidays came and brought something even better. I'd relaxed my sugar restriction by Thanksgiving, knowing it would only drive me crazy over the holidays. So when I went to my aunt Annette's annual pie gathering, she found me enjoying a small slice of strawberry-rhubarb pie.

She took in my new figure. "You look like you're about the size your mom was."

"I think so, or not far off."

"That's what I thought. Come with me."

Bemused, I put down my plate and followed her into the bedroom. Then I caught my breath, and my eyes filled with tears when I saw familiar clothes laid out on her bed.

"After your mom died, your dad had me go through her clothes to see if I wanted anything before he gave it away. I took these, but they don't fit very well, or the coloring doesn't work for me. I think they might fit you now, though. Why don't you try them on and see if you want them."

Once Annette left, I paused a moment to look at the two skirts and two dresses, remembering Mom wearing them, trying to wrap my mind around this new development. I tried them on, feeling as if I was becoming her, especially once I realized they fit me. One skirt felt a little snug, but I thought that would change after I achieved my goal weight. One dress, dark green with yellow geometric patterns on it, shocked me by hanging a little loose.

I modeled it for Annette, and she echoed what our relatives said at the pie party. "You look so much like your mother."

"I know."

"Do you know what happened to her jewelry?"

It seemed like a non sequitur, but I answered, "I don't think anything's happened with it. As far as I know it's all still at the house."

"Good. I gave your mom a green and gold necklace and earrings to go with the dress, so you might want to see if you can find them."

"I'll do that." I paused a moment, struggling not to break down as I gathered my thoughts. "And thank you so much for this. Right after Mom died, Dad asked if I wanted to look through her clothes, but I didn't. I never thought I'd be able to wear any of it, so I didn't see the point."

Annette gave me a hug, both of us tearing up. Of Mom's three sisters, Annette always seemed most like her, and for a moment it felt like hugging Mom.

She stepped back, smiled, and said, "You're welcome. I'm glad I could save something for you."

I drove home with a warmed heart, occasionally glancing in the rearview mirror at the clothing in my back seat, smiling but on the edge of tears.

My joy soared the next day at Dad's house. I found the earrings and necklace quickly, as well as other jewelry I wanted, but then Dad threw me for another loop.

"You know, I kept your mother's red dress, too. Do you want to see if you can wear it?"

I closed my eyes. The dress, Mom's favorite, always complemented her natural beauty. Bright red, with a print of vibrant flowers, it buttoned down the front with a V-neck and hinted at cleavage. The sides had ties to cinch it and accentuate her slender waist. The sleeves fell short but flowing, and it went down to mid-calf. I could picture her in the dress with perfect ease, but me?

"All right," I agreed in a daze.

I followed him down the hallway to the bedroom, a place I tried to avoid after Jackie's renovations turned it all pink. But the dress hanging in the closet was exactly as I remembered, a vivid reminder of earlier life.

"Here you go," he said before leaving and closing the door.

I trembled as I slid on the dress. As it settled comfortably around me, I had the sense of slipping into Mom's skin. I knew some women complained about becoming like their mothers, but I didn't mind. I wanted to keep her as alive as I could.

I walked into the kitchen, and Dad looked at me for a long moment before saying in a thick voice, "It fits."

"I didn't know if it would, but I'm glad."

"So am I." He paused again. "Wow. You do look like her."

"Thank you." How strange to think of me as beautiful. I couldn't help wondering if, like Mom, I would turn heads while wearing her dress.

Dad must have been thinking along the same lines because he asked, "Have you thought about pursuing a relationship now?"

"I have, but not until next year. I still have a little more weight I want to lose."

I didn't mention my fear of being attractive. I had avoided thinking much about it after my initial sense of panic, and I wanted to keep it in the closet, at least for now.

After I changed back into my regular clothes and returned to the kitchen, we talked a little more about my weight loss. My jaw dropped when he said, "I've been thinking about this a lot, and I want to tell you, your mother and I should never have bugged you about your weight. I'm sorry we did."

I gasped. Dad didn't talk much about emotions, or admit wrongdoing, although he had become more open since Mom's death.

When he said it, something inside me shifted, as if a huge weight had rolled off my shoulders, a burden I had grown so accustomed to carrying that I didn't notice it except by its absence. For the first time in a long while, I felt like I might have a real relationship with my father. It made me smile.

With tears in my eyes again, I gave him a hug. "Apology accepted," I finally said. "And thank you for saying that. It means a lot."

"I only wish I had realized it sooner." He returned my hug, his own eyes suspiciously moist.

I left feeling more peaceful and joyful than I had since Mom died. I should have known such happiness couldn't last.

16 Endings

January 2003 to March 2003—age 26, 135 pounds and losing

January 1, 2003

Back in 1991, when I said I was going to try to lose weight, my goal was between 120–125, which is also my goal now. It's interesting because when I started this process a little over two years ago, my goal was 140, then it dropped to 130, and then to 120-ish. The good news is, this time I'm actually going to get there.

The first blow fell at the beginning of the year. While taking a shower, I leaned over to get the shampoo and unthinkingly glanced down.

I had loose skin on my chest.

I started shaking. How long had this been a problem? Was it because of my more recent restriction? I didn't know, but it made me nervous and bitter, since part of my decision to lose weight slowly had been to avoid this. I had always thought of myself looking like Mom, with her smooth and unwrinkled skin, never considering it might not be the case for me.

Once out of the shower I steeled myself for a closer look. Loose skin also wrinkled my stomach and legs and arms. Between that, stretch marks, and myriad scars, I seemed monstrous all over again. Disheartened and cheated, I quickly dressed, not wanting to confront my image anymore. I didn't remember anyone ever saying that losing weight might not be enough to reach my ideal.

The discovery made me ease up on my restrictive eating and revise my goal: to reach 125 by the end of March and stop there. Having a defined end point relieved me, even if I didn't like the cause.

More bad news arrived on Saturday, January 11, 2003 while Shelly and I played cribbage at my kitchen table. The phone rang, and when I answered it, Dad's leaden tone immediately alerted me to something going on.

"Hi Erica. I have some bad news. Jackie left me."

My stomach dropped. Despite my reservations about how soon Jackie had come into our lives and some of the ways she openly criticized Dad, he had been happier with her, and Marie had also become very attached to her. I had finally started accepting this as the new way of life, but apparently no more.

"I'm so sorry."

"Would you be able to come over? Jeremiah's already on his way, and it would be easier to talk to both of you at the same time."

"Of course. I'll be there as soon as I can."

"What happened?" Shelly asked after I hung up. When I told her, she said, "I'll go with you."

I drove to the house in a daze, uncertain how to react. Seeing Dad, looking abruptly old and defeated, quickly made me realize I wanted him to be happy, even as dismayed as I had been by his early dating. My heart ached for him, and Jeremiah, Shelly and I had to coax him out of his depression enough to eat something when we took him out for dinner.

I talked to him again the next day, and he seemed to be adjusting as well as possible. My fears for his wellbeing subsided a little by Monday, and I went into work eager to hear Thea's take on the situation.

Until the layoffs started.

Thea got her notice first. When she told me, after a moment of shock I gave her a hug and said, "Oh, God, Thea, I'm so sorry. Do you know why they let you go?"

She shrugged, shoulders going sharply up and down as she collected her things. "The company needs to make some changes."

Then the phone rang. I had to answer it, somehow try to do my job and deal with customer support issues without letting my voice crack. I ended the call as soon as I could, watching as more people went down to the office. Every time someone came back, I waited, paralyzed, to see who went next, and I hated myself a little for my relief when they didn't call for me.

Finally the ordeal ended. I slowly made the rounds of goodbyes, still in some denial. These people had seen me through Mom's death, Dad's marriage, my weight loss and resulting transformation. I felt like I had lost my secondary family.

In the midst of sorrow, I received a precious gift. One of the men being let go gave me a big hug and said, "You look beautiful. I hope you don't lose too much more weight."

I barely managed to get out, "Thank you." I returned to my desk, crying.

No man outside of my family had ever called me beautiful.

For that matter, I couldn't remember when a man *in* my family had said it. Although I still didn't think of myself as beautiful, especially after discovering the loose skin. His compliment solidified my decision not to lose more than another ten pounds.

It also gave me the last nudge of self-confidence I needed to try for a new goal, something I wouldn't have considered at a heavier weight. "I'm going to look for another job," I told Dad a couple of days later.

"I wondered whether you would. Do you have any leads?"

"Someone else who left recently told me they're hiring at her company, so I'll check it out first."

I landed an interview and an offer from my friend's company in almost no time. After I gave my notice to my manager in February, I had the sense of what it might be like to attend my own funeral. Everyone told me how wonderful I was at my job, and how sorry they would be to see me go. Some people tried to convince me to stay, but I had made up my mind. I appreciated their desire to keep me on, but I knew it would be too different and difficult to continue in the same place without many of the people who had supported and befriended me.

The decision made me realize how I had changed in terms of self-confidence. Even with my loose skin, I had become comfortable with myself.

That became clearer not long after, as I wrote in my journal:

March 7, 2003

This morning I woke from an extremely odd dream in which I was walking around outside an office building wearing only underwear, and I was trying to get up to the third floor to get a sweater without being seen, but there were too many people around. To my knowledge, that's the first naked (mostly) dream I've ever had, and I have to wonder about the correlation with my weight loss. Before, I couldn't bear to look at myself clothed, let alone naked, so I had no visual for a dream—but now I do.

As icing on the cake, I received an e-mail from Dad with a surprise in it. He wrote, "I wanted to let you know that I'm very proud of you, and your mother would have been, too. She would have been telling everyone at school about you."

I started crying as I wrote back, because of the compliment, and thinking how I had finally lost weight the way Mom had always hoped. Sadly, she couldn't be part of it.

As I wrote in my journal:

But I guess it means that I'm doing the right thing, doing what would make her proud and happy even though she'll never know. It doesn't stop me from missing her, though.

It reminded me I still had one more goal related to my weight: climbing Katadhin again and scattering her ashes from the summit.

17 Lifting the Spell

Spring and Summer 2003—age 27, 125 pounds

March 16, 2003

I've been thinking a lot about change, and how it appears in our lives, and what constitutes the most significant change. Certainly things like marriage, birth, death, new jobs, new homes are all very life-altering, but I almost wonder if the changes that creep up on us unawares are perhaps not the more significant. Mom died, and that changed all our lives—for me, it triggered my weight loss. That was a deliberate decision, stubbornly stuck to, and yet when I began I had no idea of the other changes that would accompany it. I think of myself three years ago, starting to prepare for the memorial service, and I don't think that younger me would recognize who I've become as her future self.

And I don't only mean the physical changes, but everything else that has come along with it: confidence, actual positive self-esteem, ability to look a stranger in the eye, and smile and say hello, willingness to try new things, sociability, etc. I was thinking about this some at book group and realized that I could actually hang out with a group of familiar and unfamiliar people and enjoy myself, that I might actually be making friends, that all these other people are interested in my life. So very, very strange. I think of how insular I was, and how I never wanted to vary my routine, and how I felt somehow superior in my solitary suffering (the alliteration slipped in of its own accord), like I was special and unique in feeling lost and alone.

But of course that's not true. Three other members of the group are also motherless, as no doubt are many others; other people have suffered far worse than the burden of being an overweight, bespectacled, intelligent adolescent with furtive dreams of publication. Which is not to say that I'm not unique, because we all are, but I think I would do better focusing on commonalities more than differences.

And at least I've changed enough to recognize this about myself, a change that is at least as significant as the weight loss and dedication that triggered it. So I wonder, have I finally, finally emerged from my chrysalis to fly free in the world, as I conjectured so long ago now (almost 7 years)? Does the butterfly remember that time of transition, or what it was like to be a caterpillar?

About the butterfly I don't know, but for me, I feel that road to freedom no longer beckons me from some distant place, shimmering and enticing as a mirage of the sea, but rather that it has now deposited me at the next step on my path, a familiar and dear presence at my back, urging me on. Whence from here, I cannot say, only that my heart is light with hope.

At my book group meeting in March, we started talking a little about weight, and one of the women asked, "Do you mind if I ask you a personal question?"

I shook my head. "Go ahead."

"Have you noticed changes in how you're treated since losing weight?"

I hadn't thought much about the question. "It's hard to say," I said finally. "I think people do treat me differently. They're friendlier and more helpful, but I don't know if it's my perception of others that's changed, or my perception of myself, and how much is because of improved confidence. It's hard to pinpoint."

Thoughts about how people saw me came up again on Easter, when Jeremiah asked over dinner, "How's the new job? It's been, what, about a month?"

"Yes, and it's going pretty well. I'm still learning, but the people seem very nice and helpful."

"Are you glad you left your old job?" Dad asked.

I considered. "Mostly yes. It turns out there are problems at the new company, too, but the money is good."

"That always helps. Is there anything you really miss?"

I answered with a bit of embarrassment, "Yeah. Only one person there knows I used to be heavy, so the others aren't impressed by my new size, and I don't get the compliments anymore. I didn't think I'd miss it, but I do."

I hadn't realized until the compliments stopped how much I'd grown to expect them, and relied on them for rejuvenation during the hard times of losing weight. Though I didn't plan to lose more, I wondered if the lack of admiration would make it harder to maintain my lower weight.

"Well, I think you look wonderful, and I'm glad you were able to lose so much in a sustainable way, and keep it off," Patrice said.

I had to smile. "Thanks."

"And do you think you'll get to the top of Katahdin this year?" Dad asked.

"Definitely."

I refused to even consider the possibility of another failure. To prevent it, I found a way to prepare for the hike: going up and down my stairs while listening to energetic music. I started with ten minutes at a time, then worked up to twenty-five minutes, before starting to add a weighted backpack. I didn't completely enjoy it, but it made me stronger. By July, I could do twenty-five minutes of stairs with a twenty-pound backpack, and I knew I had never been in better shape.

When we went to Baxter State Park on July 12, I had high confidence. Unfortunately, some aspects of the trip fell outside my control, such as where we stayed. I had tried to get a series of lean-tos at Roaring Brook for our group, but the availability didn't line up with our dates. Instead we stayed in the bunkhouse, which gave Dad's snores ample space to echo. Between snores, and eating too much for supper, I did not sleep well the night before the hike.

I got up at 5:30 the next morning, bleary and queasy. Dad emerged around the same time, and I told him, "We are never doing the bunkhouse again. You snore so loudly."

He grinned. "Moi? I didn't hear a thing."

I muttered and went to the outhouse while he started breakfast.

We had a large hiking group—me, Shelly, Jeremiah, our friend Sarah from Northeastern, Clara from church, and Clara's friend Jen. Luckily everyone woke early enough for us to finish eating and head out by 7:00.

Some of the group planned to go up Saddle Trail via Chimney Pond, then descend via Hamlin Ridge, but I refused to overcommit again. I didn't need to make an extra-long day of it, and Sarah had agreed to go back down Saddle with me if I wanted. I had a very simple goal: climb to the top while enjoying the journey.

I grew nervous as we started out, finding it more difficult than I expected. My feet dragged, and breakfast weighed heavily in my stomach. My breath came harder and faster than it should have given all my preparation. It dredged up my youthful embarrassment as people older and with heavier packs than me stepped jauntily past. What must they think of me? Maybe I should be glad that of our large group, only Sarah stayed with me while the others sprang ahead. The fewer people who saw my weakness, the better.

After forty-five minutes of doubt and worry and upset stomach, something changed, as if someone flipped a switch. I looked around with new alertness and realized I felt good, no longer winded or feverish, and my legs seemed strong and capable. The phrase "hitting your stride" sank in. Relieved, optimistic, and eager, I charged on with confidence.

I could finally engage in more conversation. "I'm amazed everyone else could still go on so fast even though they must have all heard Dad's snoring."

"Well, Clara's like a goat," Sarah said. "She can bound anywhere. Me, I'm a turtle, slow and steady."

I laughed. "Then I must be a tortoise."

"There's no reason for us to keep up, is there?"

"No," I admitted. "As long as we get there."

We joined the others at Chimney Pond, two hours later. The timeless beauty around us delighted me, the views lifting my heart. Enjoying the scenery allowed me to let go the bitterness of lagging behind.

It also meant I could smile at Shelly when she asked, "How are you doing?"

"Great!"

Sarah and I took a few minutes to drink and rest, and I refilled my water bottle. "So you're doing okay?" Clara asked as she came to sit next to me, long legs stretched out before her, short curly hair ruffling in the wind.

I knew she meant more than the physical. "Yeah, so far. It helps that I haven't been thinking too much."

"Good idea. Over-thinking gets you in trouble." Her brown eyes twinkled; like me, she was a self-confessed over-analyzer.

"Hey guys, we should probably get going." Jeremiah pointed at the sky darkening in the distance. "Those don't look like friendly clouds."

I nodded. "Right." I spared one regretful look back as we moved out, wishing we could stay longer in that idyllic spot. We had a little over two more miles to go, much harder than the ascent so far.

The Saddle Trail started easily, but even so Sarah and I fell to the rear. "There they go," I said, glancing up ahead.

"Goats," she reminded me.

"Yeah. And this is definitely goat territory."

I stared at the sharply inclined trail, strewn with enormous boulders left by the glaciers eons ago. I thought about how some people never questioned their ability to climb mountains, how they simply knew their bodies would be up for the challenge. I realized it would never be the case for me, but at least all my preparation paid off. Despite the effort, I enjoyed much of the climb and didn't feel nearly as tired as the year before.

At last we came within sight of the next milestone, the plateau. "I think this is the worst part," I said, eyeing the steep remaining pitch with resignation. "See all the pink stuff?" Sarah nodded. "That's loose shale, and it can be slippery going."

"Okay. So we'll go slow." Seeing my expression, she grinned back. "Well, slower."

We went carefully and made it without serious mishap, only a few slips and slides. I crested the ledge of the plateau with a surge of joy. I knew, now, I would make it.

We found everyone else waiting on the ledge. "You guys doing okay?" Jeremiah asked.

"Yes. You?"

"We're good, just a little chilly."

As he said it, the wind cut through my clothes, and I shivered. It took me a minute to put on my jacket, and I watched enviously as Sarah zipped pant legs onto the bottom of her shorts. My calves already sported goosebumps.

"Shall we?" Jeremiah asked.

He led the way, and this time we stayed together as we made the final push. I forged onward with a light heart, even though the level ground of the plateau did not mean "easy". The trail, composed of a multitude of small rocks, threatened to trip us or turn an ankle. It also didn't help when gusts whipped around us hard enough to make me clamp down on my head with my hand. I couldn't stop shaking in my thin jacket. The enshrouding fog made it hard to tell how far we had to go.

We arrived at the peak just shy of noon. I stood before the sign, not quite sure what to think and feel. It almost didn't seem real. After all this time— seventeen years since my last time up here—I had made it.

"Congratulations!" Shelly gave me a big hug. "I'm so proud of you."

"Thanks." As I hugged her back, what I had done began to sink in, and I sniffled a bit. "I wish it weren't so foggy."

As soon as I said it, I realized how much the fog bothered me. I had come all this way, done so much, and yet the clouds wreathing the peak obscured the view I longed for. I had counted on seeing the panorama again.

"You did great," Jeremiah said, also giving me a hug. "And give it a few minutes. With this wind, the clouds could clear away fast."

He had a point. While waiting, we took the opportunity to snap some pictures by the Baxter Peak sign. Smiling for the camera, my spirits lifted. The cold solidity of the stone around the sign settled me. Mom had been in this same place many times, as had countless others, all connected by a thread of love for the mountain.

As we moved away to let other hikers take pictures, a massive gust of wind swirled. Exhilarated, I grabbed my hat again. I could finally see! The clouds parted magically to reveal the world below, a gorgeous spread of earth and water and sky. I grinned from ear to ear with unabashed delight. I quickly grabbed my backpack and motioned to the others. The time had come.

"Let's go down there," I suggested, pointing to an area out of the way of other hikers.

We all trooped down and huddled in a little circle, even Jen, who didn't know me and certainly hadn't known Mom. Feeling a bit self-conscious as I dug out my poem and the ashes, I asked Jeremiah, "Do you want to say anything?"

He shook his head. "Nope. I did my bit last year; this time is for you."

I swallowed hard and nodded. Tears lurked behind my eyes. With a deep breath I read my poem, clenching the paper tightly so the wind wouldn't rip it out of my hands. When I reached the part about how other people could get to know Mom by hiking Katahdin, I started to cry but kept on.

> Those who never met you
> can still get a sense of you
> by following your determined steps
> to the top.
> It is become
> a journey of remembrance,
> of love and memory and dream,
> so that every year returning,
> I can take it all in,
> listen to wind and water and loon,
> drown in an exuberance of color,
> root myself in stone
> millions of years old –
> and know that you are always here.

I quickly swiped my eyes and nose when I finished then stood up. I very carefully moved to the edge of a rock, the drop below me immediate but not frightening. With great tenderness, I opened the film canister and let the ashes go.

"I love you, Mom," I whispered, barely able to speak.

Shelly, Clara, Sarah, and Jeremiah all gave me hugs again. "That was beautiful," Clara said. "It makes me wish I could've met her."

"Thanks. I wish you could have met her, too."

Hard as it had been, I was at peace. I had come full circle, and I knew Mom was with me on the peak as much as she ever would be anywhere. I felt as though a spell had lifted. I could finally move on.

But it left me with the question—where would I go from here?

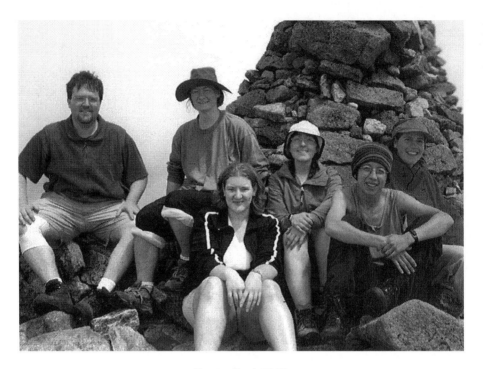

Baxter Peak 2003
Back, L–R Jeremiah, Sarah, Erica, and Jen
Front, L–R, Shelly and Clara

Part 3 Finding My Balance

18 Not the Body I Expected

Late 2003 to Summer 2004—age 27–28, 125 pounds

July 17, 2003

A few times during the hike I was totally alone, and those were dangerous moments because I started thinking about Mom. The swiftness with which grief hit me was amazing, and I literally had to stop and gasp, from sorrow not exertion, the pain was so sudden and intense.

And on the top, it was all I could do to keep things together when people told me how proud they were of me, and how proud Mom would have been. Reading the poem was wrenching and very hard to even start, let alone get through.

But scattering the ashes was more an act of closure than sorrow. It was hard in the sense that it's the closest I'll be to seeing the top with Mom, but as I wrote in the poem, now she'll always be there, at least in a way. I make no claims of what happens after death, but so long as I remember, she's still with me, and I can feel her close when I walk the same paths she took.

For a few minutes after scattering the ashes, I simply stood and took in the view. Slowly the truth sank in: I had accomplished something monumental, and Mom would have been incredibly proud of me, as proud as I was of myself. A glow of pure happiness filled me.

"We should probably head out," Jeremiah said. "Especially those of us going down Hamlin Ridge. We have quite a ways to go."

I lingered, soaking in the moment, before the cold and a desire to share my success with Dad encouraged me to move. Elated, it practically seemed I could float down the mountain, without a care for rocks or the distance we had to travel. I started towards the Saddle Trail with Sarah, smiling and at peace with the world.

My delight lasted for about ten minutes. Then, a little ahead of us, Shelly turned her ankle sharply on a rock and fell. When Sarah and I caught up with the rest of the party, Shelly stood but with a grimace of pain.

"I think I'm going back down Saddle with you," she told me, taking a tentative step.

"Will you be able to make it?" My bubble deflated as I became aware of our precarious position, the many miles between us and help. We didn't even have an ACE bandage.

"I don't have much choice, so yeah." She gave me a tight smile. "Good thing I have a high tolerance for pain."

I couldn't argue. So while Jeremiah, Clara, and Jen continued on to descend via Hamlin Ridge, Shelly, Sarah, and I went down Saddle.

As we started out, I alternated watching my footing and monitoring Shelly. Worried as I was, I knew I couldn't do anything about her injury, and that constantly asking how she felt wouldn't help. I bit my tongue and pressed on.

Relief came a short time later when I saw a young woman in a khaki Baxter State Park uniform coming up the trail. I had never been happier to see a park ranger.

We stopped and sat to wait for her. She arrived a few minutes later, cheerful and chipper despite carrying a backpack nearly as big as her. "Hello," she said with a friendly smile. "How are you ladies doing?"

"Not the best," Shelly answered. "I hurt my ankle on the top just as we started back."

"I'm sorry to hear that. Do you want an ACE bandage to wrap around it? Or I think I have an air cast." I breathed a sigh of gratitude. Help hadn't been so far after all.

"The air cast would be great," Shelly said. The ranger found it quickly, and when Shelly stood after putting it on, she looked relieved. "That definitely helps, thanks."

"Good. I hope you have an easier time the rest of the way."

We continued, Shelly obviously feeling better as she moved more easily and started chatting. I stopped worrying and focused on the hike, wanting to enjoy the descent and savor my success.

Until my knees started hurting.

At first it didn't seem serious, an occasional twinge of pain on a long step down. Then the twinges came more frequently. The problem intensified to the point where each step brought pain like knives stabbing into my kneecaps.

I blinked back tears and tried to breathe through it. How ridiculous! Here Shelly had seriously injured her ankle but didn't complain, and I hadn't done a thing but wanted to fall in my tracks and cry.

Instead of stopping I slowed down, moving gingerly as I sought out approaches requiring the least impact. Sarah must have noticed because she asked, "Are you all right?"

I shook my head, a quick, jerky motion. "My knees are bothering me a lot, which is weird because that didn't happen last year, and I weigh less now."

"That is weird. If it's really bad, you could try going down sideways. I've heard that helps some people."

With nothing to lose, I tried. To my surprise it helped, enough for me to finish the hike without complete agony. Even so, by the time we limped back to the lean-to's, my triumphant moment at the top seemed like a long time ago.

"Did you make it?" Dad asked.

"Yeah."

"Congratulations! I'm proud of you." He gave me a hug.

His obvious enthusiasm made me smile and revived some of my own joy as I returned his hug. "Thanks. The way up was actually pretty great, and I read my poem and scattered Mom's ashes. Coming down, though, wasn't as good. We have some casualties."

We shared stories in the evening, and at least none of the group who took the Hamlin Ridge trail had any problems. The next morning we headed home as early as possible, so Shelly could get some ice on her ankle and keep her foot elevated for a while.

After a couple of days, though, her mom and boyfriend convinced her she should also go to a doctor. She called to tell me the results.

"Turns out I fractured my ankle."

"You hiked down on a broken ankle?" I couldn't believe it.

"Yeah. Like I said, high tolerance for pain. The good news is my boyfriend is being really sweet about it and helping me carry stuff, since being on the third floor isn't very convenient. But how are your knees doing?"

"Better, although they still twinge sometimes on stairs. I'm taking it easy and hoping it clears up soon."

Within a few days my knees seemed mostly recovered, just as well since I soon had other things to worry about. I called Dad in some shock to tell him, "I got laid off."

"Oh my god," he said. "And you weren't there very long!"

"Four months." I shook my head. "But it wasn't just me. They hired a bunch of us, thinking they'd have more sales, and they didn't. At least they gave me a good severance package, and people at my old company already said I could go back if I want."

I appreciated the offer to return to my old company, but it also gave me pause. I decided to hold off on a decision for a few weeks and instead enjoy the summer in Maine. That included picking blueberries with Jeremiah and

Marie, something I discovered I loved, and visiting state parks with Clara, who had the summer off.

On one of our visits, I asked Clara about something I'd been considering for a while: "Do you know when and where the Farmers' Market is held?"

"Wednesday mornings it's in Monument Square, and Saturday mornings at Deering Oaks Park. Are you thinking of going?"

"Yeah, I'd like to do more cooking. I've mostly been eating the same things for the last three years, because once I found something that worked for losing weight, I didn't want to jinx it by eating anything else. Now I'm tired of that and want to experiment. Plus, I'm eating a lot more these days, so it seems like a good time to branch out."

"What do you mean you're eating more?"

"It's strange, but since I'm not trying to lose weight, it takes more food for me to maintain, especially because I still exercise a lot."

I didn't say how much more I ate, finding it both astonishing and almost embarrassing. After all my struggles with weight, how could I possibly eat so much and not gain? For the first time, I felt sympathy for people who had metabolisms so high they had to eat constantly to prevent being underweight.

Clara nodded. "That makes sense. Let me know if you want to go to the market together or talk about cooking ideas."

"Thanks. I might take you up on that, once I figure out what I like to eat now. That's the other problem. My tastes have changed so much I can't always be sure how I'll react to things."

The difference in taste became even clearer when I went to the Farmers' Market early Saturday. With the morning sun catching the mist and streaming through the tall, majestic trees, Deering Oaks Park had a slightly magical and ethereal air. The food impressed me even more. The farmers presented what looked like a giant cornucopia of bountiful delights, including many things I had never tried. Eggplant? Kale? Rainbow chard? Heirloom tomatoes? New varieties of apples, like ginger gold and honey crisp? And who knew peaches and plums grew in Maine? Cucumbers only four for a dollar? A revelatory experience, with possibilities both overwhelming and enticing.

Looking at it all, I recognized the feeling I used to have in candy stores, wanting to try everything. Except this time, I hungered for fruits and vegetables. Drawn to them, I knew they would not only taste good but would keep my body feeling good. Given the choice between this and a candy store, I'd now choose this. Going home with bags full of veggies and a light heart, I marveled at my change of attitude.

I enjoyed experimenting with the new foods back home, but much as I liked having the extra free time for outings and cooking, by the end of August I needed to decide about work. After some thought, I chose to go back to my old company, but to a different department, knowing that returning to Customer

Support would be too difficult with so many familiar faces missing. My increased self-confidence helped, allowing me to believe I could try something new, and I looked forward to my role as a business analyst.

I also secretly hoped my return would trigger renewed compliments related to my weight loss. It didn't happen. It disappointed me, but it made sense. Now at a stable, steady weight, people would no longer have a reason to focus on my size. I only wished someone had told me maintaining might not be exciting.

I reminded myself I had not lost weight to please anyone else or earn compliments. I had done it for me, to be able to accomplish things I couldn't have before, like my climb up Katahdin. I could appreciate it more now when my knees didn't often bother me, and I looked for other ways of enjoying my lighter body, noticing the smaller things like easily fitting into the bus seat with another person and my discovery of new foods.

Unfortunately, another problem I'd encountered some time before hadn't corrected itself as I'd hoped. I no longer had my period. I stopped thinking about compliments and instead worried about my health.

While such a change might thrill some women, I knew it meant something had gone wrong in my body, and after almost nine months, I doubted my cycle would spontaneously resume. This alarmed me much more than the loose skin or knee issues because it hit on something I'd only truly appreciated since Mom's death: I wanted children.

Thinking about that, after starting work again in September, I finally made an appointment to look into the problem. "I haven't had my period since last November, and I'm wondering if it's related to my weight loss," I told the doctor.

"What do you mean about your weight? How much did you lose?" she asked. I explained my situation, and she nodded. "It's not uncommon for women who have lost so much body fat to experience this, what we call hypothalamic amenorrhea. If you think about it, you lost a whole person, and to your body, that feels like trauma. My suggestion is to have you go on the pill for six to twelve months. It might help reset your system, and the hormones will help protect your bones."

While relieved to know this wasn't completely unusual, I noticed the doctor's uncertainty about recovery. "You said the pill might help. How likely is it?"

"Eighty percent of women regain their cycles."

I started to panic. "Meaning twenty percent don't. And if I fall into that twenty percent, then what? What else could I try? Does it mean I can't have kids?"

She gave me a reassuring smile. "First, don't worry about children. There's no reason you wouldn't be able to conceive, with some help. And if your body doesn't resume its cycle, I could send you to a reproductive endocrinologist, although I'm not aware of any way of triggering your hormones to start up again. But odds are you won't have to worry about that."

I took the prescription and went home with a sinking feeling in my stomach. I wanted to believe the pill would help, but I knew numbers well enough to realize twenty percent meant one in five, a large margin. I tried not to obsess about it. I could do nothing but wait and see.

My body had betrayed me, though. Here I had lost all this weight, which everyone had assured me would be a good thing, and now this, on top of the other problems I'd had. I always thought being thin would automatically make me healthier in every way, but clearly it didn't. I couldn't help remembering that Mom had also been thin, and it hadn't saved her.

I fought off bitterness, instead settling into my new routines of work and cooking and church and social events. I managed to forget about some of my health concerns in the fun, particularly with certain church activities.

Jeremiah, Clara, a few others and I had started holding evening, lay-led worship services in an attempt to attract more people our own age to church. We had such a good time, though, it often seemed we did it as much for ourselves as anyone else.

I especially liked sharing the results of my cooking and baking experiments at the services, since we knew offering food would appeal to young adults. It also allowed me to indulge what remained of my sweet tooth. I enjoyed the same warm sense of community I'd had when baking during my earlier days working at Draper.

At first I struggled with guilt about bringing sugary and fatty foods like brownies and cookies and cupcakes, when I didn't eat them as much anymore. To appease my sense of culpability, I made sure we included options with more nutritional content and stopped worrying about it.

I also enjoyed my new position at work, finding I liked the necessary attention to detail and thinking about software design. I started finding a balance with everything, and then in early 2004, the company moved to a new office on the sixth floor of a nearby building.

Up until then, I hadn't done much to stress my knees, but once in the new location, I decided to try taking the stairs. Going up five levels would give me a decent workout, and going down would be a good test for my knees.

Descending the first flight went fine, but on the second flight, the pain started. By the time I reached the third floor, the knife-like stabbing had returned with a vengeance, so strong I simply couldn't continue. I had to take the elevator the rest of the way down, fighting tears the whole way.

Worse, my knees didn't recover. After a few weeks, even a few steps triggered the stabbing pain. Then my hips developed a constant ache. I started walking very slowly, nearly hobbling at times, feeling crippled when I tried to stand after sitting for a long time and almost couldn't make it.

I wanted to cry. At least before, even with the other health problems, I'd been able to enjoy my new size and level of ability. Now I had all I could do to climb the stairs in my condo, sometimes needing to pause between each step. I hated it, hated knowing I had never had these problems while heavy. Other issues, sure, but nothing that prevented me from taking a walk.

"It's so awful," I told Clara. "I feel like I'm eighty instead of twenty-seven."

"I'm sorry. That's no fun. Have you gone to your doctor?"

"No, but I guess I should."

My doctor directed me to a physical therapist, and she only needed one look to tell me the problem. "Your kneecaps are out of alignment. They're not tracking properly when they flex, which is why you're feeling the pain. But we can start you on some exercises to strengthen the muscles around your knee, which will help stabilize the joint."

"Okay, but what about my hips?" I asked.

"It's all connected. Because of your knee problems, you're walking and carrying yourself differently, and it's affected your hips."

"Do you think I'll need surgery?" I couldn't help giving voice to my biggest fear.

"I doubt it, but you should see an orthopedic surgeon to be sure. In the meantime, let's get you going with some exercises, and you could also start taking glucosamine chondroitin."

She showed me how to do hip abductions and adductions using a resistance band, with instructions on how often to do them at home. Then a few days later I met with the orthopedic surgeon.

After I explained the situation, I added, "And it's very ironic to have knee problems after losing weight, instead of while heavy. Do you think the weight loss could be causing it?"

"It might be part of it, but there are a lot of factors," he pointed out. "Since you've lost weight, it's probably changed the way you sit, and the girth of your legs is smaller. You've lost muscle mass, but you're also probably more active, so there are multiple considerations." I nodded, recognizing the truth of that. "The main thing is to keep up the physical therapy. Surgery is the last resort, especially because there's no guarantee of success."

That sounded like a good approach to me, and as I thought about it, I realized my legs and knees had developed to carry a certain amount of weight. Now with my weight drastically different, it would probably take a while for everything to recalibrate. I only hoped it would and I could go back to appreciating my body instead of living in constant pain.

19 Control Issues

March 2004 to Early 2005—age 27–28, 125–130 pounds

March 5, 2004

It's odd when I realize these days how much I think about food. I've even started thinking about it in relation to the trip I'm taking in September to visit my friends overseas. I didn't used to be like this, keeping mental track of what and when I've eaten, and focusing on how my body feels. Before, my food issues were around hiding what and when I ate. Not doing that anymore, at least, is one good thing. But I sometimes wish I could go back and just reclaim the unconcern about what I ate, but I know I never can. It's depressing sometimes, to know I'll have to do this forever, but when I go back to pictures of myself before, or journal entries, I know it's worth it.

My knees slowly recovered over the summer of 2004, and I eagerly awaited my trip to visit my friends Nina and David. David and I planned to stay with Nina in Belgium for a few days, then I'd go back to Ireland with David to visit with him and his wife for a while longer.

Excited as I was, I worried about not having as much say over what or when I ate. I would also have to forego my morning ritual of stepping on the scale for reassurance about my weight.

When I mentioned it to my aunt Patrice, she said, "I'm sure you'll do fine. And even if you gain a couple of pounds, you'll be able to lose them pretty quickly once you get home."

I wanted to believe her, but I didn't quite trust myself. My concern dogged me steadily until I arrived in Belgium on September 22. As soon as I passed through customs, I saw Nina and David waiting for me and waved. Excitement allowed me to shake off my anxiety and tiredness.

When I reached them, Nina immediately exclaimed, "Oh my god, look at you! You sent pictures, but I didn't think you'd be this skinny!"

"Thanks," I said, smiling broadly. "You look great, too." And she did, having also lost some weight, although even when she'd been heavier I always considered her beautiful.

"What about me?" David asked. "Don't I look grand?"

Nina flapped her hand dismissively. "You just look the same."

We all laughed—it seemed like no time had passed since we last visited.

We quickly settled in, catching up on recent life events. This included telling them about my knee problems, since I needed Nina's help finding a place to do my exercises with the resistance band.

David asked, "Are your knees still bothering you a lot? You seem to be walking okay."

"I'm better, but not completely recovered. The exercises help, but I think I've done as much as I can with those, so I may start going to a gym to have access to a leg press. At least I could hike a smaller mountain at Baxter State Park this summer without too much trouble. I had to wear knee braces, but it was still a lot better."

I left out how embarrassed I'd been when buying the braces. I tried regular ones at CVS, only to discover they wouldn't fit over the bulk of my lower thighs, even with the weight loss. In the end I had to visit a medical store for special, strap-on braces. I pushed the memory away, wanting to focus on the positive.

We spent a lot of time at Nina's apartment over the next few days, catching up and enjoying each other's company, with a few outings for a change of scenery. During it all, I paid close attention to my hunger and eating, partly because of weight concerns but more because I wanted to avoid being overly hungry or stuffing myself to the point of discomfort. As a result, I often opted for salads as a main course when we ate out, knowing that way I'd have room for dessert or a side dish if I wanted more.

I held to this pattern on our day trip to Bruges. It meant salad for two meals, lunch and dinner. At dinner, Nina looked at me oddly and asked, "Don't you get tired of salads?"

"Not often. Besides, we did have that chocolate earlier, and I'll probably get dessert."

I didn't think much of the comment, simply enjoyed myself on the rest of the trip, including my longer visit to Ireland. Nina, though, must have dwelt a lot more on my eating habits. After I returned home, I didn't hear from her for months, even to acknowledge my e-mails or the photo book I sent her of the trip. I began worrying, wondering if she was okay.

She finally responded in January 2005, and the explanation for her silence caught me completely off-guard.

She had hesitated writing, not knowing how to tell me about her surprise and agitation at seeing how I had changed. She said I "criticized everything and enjoyed nothing" because I was "controlled and uptight." I had become "rigid and unyielding," both in how I thought and the way I communicated. It reminded her of her own earlier control issues, and she offered to share how she changed some of those things. She worried my behavior would drive people away from me, and I deserved better.

Incredulous, I stared at the computer screen. Then denial gave way to pain. Sliding out of my chair, I curled up on the floor. I sobbed for what might have been forever, shaking badly, my stomach tight with knots. I could hardly breathe. I came close to wanting my heart to stop, simply to ease the hurt.

The e-mail brought back all my old fears and anguish about rejection, but this time all the worse because I hadn't expected them to surface again. I'd thought losing weight would prevent this type of thing, not cause it.

I didn't question the truth of Nina's statements. I simply accepted them at face value. After all, no one could deny I had changed, and I took her word the change had been for the worse. Yet she liked me before. What had I lost aside from weight? Anguished, I turned to write in my journal, my tears blotting some of the words:

> The worst part of this, though, is that the person she describes and apparently saw does not sound like someone anyone would want to be friends with. And I don't want to be that person. But maybe I am. I don't want to be alone, but I am, and I wonder—is it because I've driven everyone away by the way I am? That possibility hurts so damn much, and I can't stop crying because of it. Then again, maybe that's good— that's another area where I'm sometimes too controlling. I just really want someone to give me a hug and tell me they love me—but I'm by myself.

Eventually I cried myself out. Drained on many levels, I attempted to do other things, but I couldn't focus. Nina's e-mail haunted me. Then Shelly called and I told her about it, inwardly afraid she would confirm everything.

I drooped in relief when she said in surprise, "Really? I wouldn't say that. I do think you've changed, but for the better."

Her affirmation reminded me of all the people who had commented on positive changes in my personality, saying I had become happier and friendlier. I also realized David hadn't echoed Nina, and I'd visited with him longer.

Clutching the shreds of my self-confidence, I gathered my courage and asked other people if they agreed with Nina.

"Actually, I think you're less controlling now," Jeremiah said. "You don't seem as focused on details or planning. You said she's had weight problems, too. Maybe in some ways she's jealous of you, and this is how it's coming out."

I hadn't even considered that, but Dad agreed with him. "Usually when people react too strongly, it's very close to home for them, and something they're trying to deal with. And the only times when I notice you being controlling at all is around food." It reminded me how Nina had commented on her own control issues.

Other people replied in a similar way, but David's response helped the most. He said I didn't seem particularly different, apart from one day when I appeared a little extra focused on food.

My mood improved. I hadn't become a horrible person. I still had friends, people who loved me as I was. But Nina had a point, at least in part. I knew I focused a lot on food issues, including worrying what people would think when they saw me eat because now I had an image to maintain after losing weight.

I also realized Nina and I first met in college, before Mom's death, before I had any major responsibilities. Now I had to work, pay a mortgage, and live with the reality of mortality, loss, and grief. All of it had an impact.

I wrote back to Nina with some of my thoughts, but after a few exchanges, punctuated by increasingly long gaps, we fell out of touch. I couldn't forget how she saw me, and how her view made me feel badly about myself. I did the only thing I could: consider my behavior more closely, and try to be more relaxed and open.

It helped, but I soon realized my life changes impacted more than my friendships. They also played a large part in my dating adventures.

20 The Dating Game

Spring 2004 to Fall 2005—age 28–29, 125–130 pounds

August 14, 2004

I just finished The Time Traveler's Wife, *and I noticed how much sex there was in it. And I wonder, even now, if anyone would actually want to sleep with me, with my stretch marks and loose skin, and if so would it be anyone I'd want to sleep with.*

I've also been thinking about how strange it is that I've never been in a relationship. It can't help but make me wonder at times what's wrong with me, and despair of ever learning all these things that everyone else knows.

Shortly after losing weight, I'd been at loose ends, wondering what to do with myself. I decided I needed a new goal: finding a boyfriend.

I quickly realized I had no idea how to navigate this unfamiliar territory. How would I explain my earlier weight issues to a date? What if it scared him off? Would I even feel comfortable discussing all that?

I thought it might help to start by sharing my history in a safe place. The perfect opportunity came in April 2004 when Jeremiah, Clara, a couple of others and I organized an evening worship service for church with a theme of Food.

During one of our planning meetings at my place, I said, "I'd like to share some of my own experiences with food and weight, if that's okay."

Clara grabbed a Dove dark chocolate from my stash. "Sounds like a great idea."

"And we should ask Dad if he'll make bread for it," Jeremiah said.

"I'll ask him," I said.

I had an ulterior motive in offering. I wanted to let Dad know what I'd be sharing and tell him, "I wanted to warn you—you might get mentioned during my piece."

"Okay, consider me warned," he said.

"Do you want to read it beforehand?"

"No, I'll take it as it comes."

On the evening of the service, my turn came after the opening readings. I stood and focused on the chalice flickering in the center of the circle, remembering no one came here to judge me. I drew a deep breath and began.

I didn't look up much as I gave the three-minute version of my story: the focus on my weight and eating, my obsession with sweets, my feeling that nothing mattered as long as I was heavy, my decision to lose weight after Mom's death, my process of shrinking and now maintaining.

As I spoke, I worried Dad might think I meant to attack him or point fingers, when I only wanted to share my perspective. I had to wait until the end of the service to find out how he took it, but first a lot of other people came up to me.

Some said how much they liked the service. Even more said, "I had no idea you struggled with weight! Congratulations on losing it."

What strange feedback. My weight had been such a central, defining part of my life, and yet anyone meeting me now would never know how being so heavy made me anguished and bitter.

Dad, though, knew my earlier self all too well, although we didn't get a chance to talk until the potluck started. When he approached me, I didn't know what to expect, but certainly not what he said.

"Good service. And as far as what you read, I want to apologize." I stared at him as he continued, "I'm sorry for my part in making you feel that way about food and about yourself. But your mother and I were worried about you."

I blinked hard and gave him an awkward, one-armed hug while balancing my plate of food. "Apology accepted." The moment made sharing my experience in public entirely worthwhile, nerve-wracking as it had been.

It also gave me confidence in the idea of telling a potential date about my experiences. I had plenty of other concerns, though.

How would I know if someone liked me? What type and amount of physical contact would my date expect? How should I respond if I received any unwelcome advances? When should I mention my earlier weight issues and my lack of dating experience? What would I do if he rejected me because of the telltale signs of weight left on my body? How could I tell if he was interested in more than sex? When would I tell him my mom had died? What was I even looking for?

Having never dated before—I didn't count Chris—I felt like a teenager all over again, only in many ways worse. At least as a teen, no one necessarily expects you to be very experienced, but by twenty-eight?

I went on a few dates through online sites in 2004, but with no success. I put dating on hold during the end of the year, but in the spring of 2005, everything conspired to remind me of my single status. Dad had met a very nice woman named Jan online, Shelly got engaged, and I found out Marie's mom Natalie would be getting remarried. Love seemed to be in the air, so I decided to try again.

After putting up a new online profile, I didn't receive as many messages as Shelly had in her attempts, but I did meet Jared, a nice, cute guy who had a job, liked my writing, and played guitar. We made it through two dates without major issue. My hope rose.

For our third date we went for a long walk at Pineland Farms, and I decided to bite the bullet. I told him about my weight history then waited anxiously for his response.

"You lost that much weight on your own? That's amazing!"

I had half-expected rejection. The effusive compliment made me blush, but I wasn't about to complain. "Thanks."

We went back to Jared's apartment, where he made a dinner of salmon, bread with olive oil, and green beans. Then things started to go wrong.

We ate around seven, later than usual for me. Between the timing and our long walk, I needed a lot of food, except I didn't eat much. He didn't have a lot, but also, I had confessed to him about losing weight. How could I now eat ravenously in front of him? All my old insecurities rushed back, and I worried he would judge me by what I ate. At the end of the meal I remained desperately hungry. Miserable with myself, I put my dish in the sink.

Then Jared put his hands on my arms and acted like he planned to kiss me. My stomach clamored for more food, so demanding I could barely concentrate on him. If he kissed me, I'd have to stay a while longer, and then when would I be able to eat my fill? Plus, I'd seen plenty of sitcoms and references to the "third date"—would Jared expect more than kissing? I didn't think I could deal with that conversation as well, particularly not when so hungry. I ducked my head away.

"I should be going," I said, really thinking, *I need to eat.*

It embarrassed me, but I didn't know what else to do. Only after the fact, when he drifted away, did I consider how it must have looked to him. I realized I still had a ways to go before integrating my past and current selves.

Then I started e-mailing a guy named Carl who lived in Massachusetts and seemed great: sensitive, intelligent, socially conscious, a good writer, spiritual, and complimentary to me. The distance gave me pause, but he offered to drive up to meet me at the Festival of Cultural Exchange in Portland. I could hardly say no, and I waited both eagerly and nervously.

Due to some bad traffic he arrived late, by which point I'd already had a little something to eat. I figured I'd get something else small with him, assuming he'd want lunch by the time we met at 1:30.

"No, I'm okay," he said. "I tend to only have a meal at supper and a snack or two during the day. Since I had a shake for breakfast and a snack earlier, I don't need anything right now. Maybe later."

I had all I could do not to stare in both disbelief and dismay. It had never occurred to me to specify "eats regular meals" as a dating requirement. Did he not care about food? How could he not eat on a regular basis? Coming from my family with Hobbit-like tendencies to eat at almost any time, I couldn't grasp that.

"Okay," I said, hoping I didn't sound the way I felt. Thank goodness I had already eaten something.

We had fun wandering for a while, listening to music and looking at arts and crafts from different cultures, but eventually my light meal wore off. "I might get something else to eat," I said, tentative, not sure I liked being the only one eating.

"I could use something now, too."

I exhaled a breath of silent gratitude, more comfortable at the idea of eating together. We bought veggie wraps and found some steps where we could sit and have our meal.

When we finished, he looked at me thoughtfully. "You look better, like you're really satisfied now."

I didn't know what to say. He had only met me in person that day. How could he already read me so accurately? Because he was right. My niggling edge of hunger had vanished, allowing me to relax. But I didn't know what to make of such close scrutiny, even though I likely should have expected it based on our e-mails. Would I be comfortable with such focus, and our eating differences? I had grown used to thinking of any attention being negative. Could I adjust to the concept of it being positive?

I never had a chance to find out answers to any of my questions because not long afterwards, he met someone closer to home. It gave me a lot to consider, though, about how I ate, and how I thought of myself and my eating.

I realized I had largely expected everything to fall magically into place after losing weight, like the "happily ever after" of fairy tales. I was slowly learning that incorporating such a major change into my life would not happen instantly, especially when in many ways I didn't get what I expected. The question was, could I accept the reality, or would I still try to achieve my imagined ideals?

21 Transformation

Spring 2005 to Fall 2006—age 29–31, 125–130 pounds

September 10, 2006

After finally deciding to go ahead with cosmetic surgery, I found out that the doctor doing my surgery is the same one who did Mom's reconstruction, and it makes me think about how strange cause and effect is. Mom's cancer and death leading to my weight loss leading to my surgery.

It reminds me that even though it's not a lot of me, I'm sacrificing part of myself. It's not exactly an amputation, but it's not that dissimilar, either. It's exciting but scary. If I let myself think about it too much, it's almost suffocating, but it's also encouraging to consider what it might be like afterward. I got an e-mail from a friend who said that she suspects it could be a very freeing, transformative experience for me. And I hadn't quite thought of it along those lines, but she's right. I may be very butterfly-like, emerging from my wrappings as a new self.

The first time I considered the idea of cosmetic surgery came in early 2005.

I had started going to the gym in late 2004 so I could have more exercise options for my knees, but it also highlighted another problem area: my upper arms. I knew they would never be skinny, but I had hoped for something a little smaller. Although the size didn't bother me as much as the way the flesh swayed and flapped whenever I moved my arms.

I knew some of that came from loose skin, but not how much. I decided to see if I could tighten that area on my own first. As I told Shelly, "I'm going to really focus on my arms at the gym for a year, but then, if I'm still not happy with them, I'll look at cosmetic surgery." I swallowed, somewhat ashamed to admit I might not be able to reshape my body on my own.

"Wow. That's a lot to think about, but good for you for doing what you need for yourself."

I appreciated the support, though considering surgery seemed like cheating. Even so, I thought about it more seriously in June when I went shopping for a bridesmaid's dress for Shelly's wedding. Shelly had told us six bridesmaids we could choose whatever style we wanted, as long as it came in the fabric she had picked out. As it happened I preferred the styles of the sleeveless gowns. I wavered. I couldn't bear to think about exposing my arms, especially at a wedding.

One of the other bridesmaids must have noticed my distress because she reassured me, "We're going to have wraps, too, since in October it will be too cold for sleeveless." She gave me a conspiratorial smile. "Besides, I don't think any of us are very excited to show off our arms."

It surprised me. Others were also self-conscious about their arms, including people who seemed a normal size to me? But I saw no need to argue the point. I simply chose the most appealing style, a bit baffled to end up with a sleeveless, strapless, form-fitting dress.

"We'll have to take in the bust a little to make it fit, but a size six should work," the shop's owner said, making some notes.

Her off-hand comment floored me. Me? A size six bridesmaid's dress? Had I wandered into a parallel universe?

The day became even more surreal when one of Shelly's sisters asked, "Erica, can you model this for me?"

I looked blankly at her and the dress she held. "Um, I guess, but why?"

"They don't have my size, and I want to see what it looks like when worn, and you're the smallest one here."

I looked around at the other bridesmaids. She was right. "Okay."

After I tried on her choice, I ended up posing in a number of outfits. I drove home, dazed but smiling from my brief career as a model.

Over the summer, I continued working hard on my arms at the gym. I discovered I could do push-ups! And not just the easy ones while balanced on my knees. I worked up to doing twenty to twenty-five full push-ups, unexpectedly delighted by my newfound ability.

Despite my efforts, by early 2006 I didn't notice much of a difference in the shape of my arms. I successfully ignored it until I got a second bridesmaid invitation, this time from my friend Clara. I ended up with another sleeveless dress, again one I couldn't contemplate wearing without some coverage for my arms. Patrice helped me make a shrug to wear with it, but I knew I didn't want to continue hiding myself like that forever. I started looking into cosmetic surgery.

First I had to find a reputable surgeon. What if I went under the knife of a bad one and ended up disfigured, getting infections, or worse? Thankfully my doctor knew someone reliable in the field, and I scheduled a consult in May with Dr. White. Even the act of making the appointment was a huge step. I only hoped it would turn out to be the right one.

I used the time before the consultation to make some decisions and do research. After much thought, I decided the loose skin on my chest didn't bother me enough to warrant surgery; my arms, thighs, and stomach became my areas of focus.

I looked around online and found the names of the procedures I wanted to consider: arm lifts, thigh lifts, and a tummy tuck. The arm lifts seemed pretty straightforward. Reading about thigh lifts freaked me out, though, since they ran a risk of permanent nerve or muscle damage, which could impact my mobility.

I paused. Insurance didn't cover the surgery, and I knew it would be expensive, probably around $6,000 for each operation. Was vanity worth that? But then I wondered, is appearance only about vanity? Even if I accepted my body with the loose skin instead of trying to make it fit societal molds, would others accept it? Would I be judged harshly if I didn't go through with this?

With all of those conflicting thoughts roaming around my head, I didn't quite know what to feel when I went to see Dr. White, but her professionalism, good humor, and above all honesty put me at ease.

"Hold out your arms," she instructed.

I did, all too aware of the swaying skin. I needed to justify myself. "I've tried doing lots of exercises to tighten up, but it hasn't worked."

She ran her fingers along my arms then gave me a sympathetic smile. "All the exercise in the world won't change this. It's loose skin, plain and simple."

"Oh."

Her diagnosis surprised me, but it also brought instant, intense relief. I hadn't done anything wrong, and in fact I had done all I could on my own. Simply knowing that made the flaws more bearable.

She also confirmed what I had read. I would be a perfect candidate for arm lifts, with no damage apart from a scar along the inside of my arm, while work on my legs ran the risk of nerve or muscle impact. "Plus," she added, "you wouldn't even get the shape you want, since you'd still have this pouching out over your knee. You'd need liposuction for that."

I flinched inwardly. The word alone reminded me of an *X-Files* episode where liposuction went terribly wrong. I wasn't interested.

"What about my stomach?" I asked. "Would it make sense to do anything with that if I want to have kids?"

"This is another area where you'd be a perfect candidate. It would be a whole new look for you, since your torso is so lean. Even if you got pregnant, it probably wouldn't fill out all of this skin. But certainly you could wait to have that done."

After much thought, I decided I could live with my legs and my stomach, but to go ahead with my arms, the most visible area. Then I had to decide when to have the surgery, knowing I would be incapacitated for quite a while.

"I finally scheduled the surgery," I told Shelly one day when we met for lunch. "It took a long time to figure out, because I'm going to two more weddings, and I'll be traveling for work, and I want to be healed by the time we might get snow."

"So when are you having it?"

"September 13, between weddings and almost two months before I have to travel." I shook my head as I picked up a piece of melon. "I didn't realize it would be so complicated."

"You mean scheduling?"

"Everything. The problem is, I'm not supposed to drive or pick up more than five pounds for six weeks. Thank goodness I take the bus to work and can do some work from home, and at least I can walk to Rosemont Market for some groceries. But I'll need help doing laundry, and other grocery shopping, and probably cleaning the litter box. I also have follow-up doctor appointments, so I'll need rides, and because I'm going under anesthesia, someone has to be with me for twenty-four hours after the surgery to make sure I don't have a bad reaction."

She gave me a sympathetic smile. "That's a lot, but you know I'm willing to help."

"Thanks. People at church are going to do a lot, with rides and staying overnight, but if you could stop by a couple of days to help with meals and some chores, that would be great."

"Absolutely. Just let me know when you have specifics. The only thing I wouldn't be able to do is the litter box, since I'm pregnant."

I nodded. "Right. The funny thing is, that's the one thing Clara can't do, either, for the same reason. And at least once I heal up a little, I should be fine cleaning it myself. Oh, and did I tell you the ironic part?"

"What is it?"

"Two things. One, I have to buy extra-large, button down shirts because my arms will be bigger than normal at first, with swelling and because of the bandages. I can't get over needing to buy large clothing sizes again because of something I'm doing after losing weight."

She laughed. "What's the other part?"

"I'm going to deliberately overeat the night before the surgery, since I can't eat for twelve hours beforehand, and the surgery isn't scheduled until noon." I shook my head. "I keep wondering if I'm crazy to be choosing to put myself through all this. I hope it's worth it."

"You're not crazy, and I'm sure it will be worthwhile."

I appreciated her encouragement and willingness to help, and happily many others volunteered to assist. Dad and Jan promised to visit and give me some bread; Annette would also visit and bring some jam, perfect to go with the bread; Patrice offered to make some freezer-friendly meals; and other people from church, work and the neighborhood agreed to assist with transportation, groceries, and more. I hadn't realized quite how many people would be willing to help me out. I found it all very touching.

The night before the surgery, I ate a second big dinner as planned. Then, since I also couldn't drink for six hours beforehand, I got up at five in the morning to gulp over a quart of water.

In the end everything went smoothly. I came out of surgery a little woozy but otherwise fine. My arms, tightly wrapped in bandages to help prevent swelling, made me feel like a mummy, and I had to move my arms carefully due to the plastic drains taped on each side to collect fluid. I understood much better why I needed the overly large shirts.

A woman from church brought me home, and once I had settled in, she asked, "How are you feeling?"

I took inventory. "Okay. Dr. White told me I wouldn't be in much pain, since they only worked on skin and fat, not muscle."

"That's good. Do you feel up for having something to eat?"

I wasn't particularly hungry, since I had gotten some nutrients via the IV during the surgery, but I thought I should eat something. "Maybe a little soup."

She heated some up, and I gingerly used my arms, moving my spoon slowly as I ate. The tight wraps made my arms hard to bend, and I did so as little as possible. Then I went back to the couch, where we propped my arms up high on pillows to help keep the swelling down.

"I feel like such an invalid," I said.

"You may feel like one, but you seem to be doing remarkably well."

"But I can't do anything. I can't do cross stitch or braid my hair. And how can I tell the cats I can't pick them up?" I added this as Salem meowed at me from the floor, confused by all the pillows. "I knew it would be like this, but it's just odd."

We spent the rest of the evening watching a movie. Then I had to prepare for bed, which meant more pillows under my arms, making it hard to sleep and presenting an obstacle course for my other cat, Osiris, as he tried to curl up with me.

By the next morning, I decided I could safely do a little typing, so I sent out a quick e-mail to let everyone know I came through okay. The rest of the day I mostly chatted with the various people who came to keep me company and monitor my twenty-four hours after anesthesia.

I didn't have time to myself until late afternoon, when I became introspective about the whole process.

September 14, 2006

Sitting here surrounded by cats who don't understand why my lap is not available, propped up by pillows, wrapped in gauze and tapped by flexible tubing, beginning to feel greasy from lack of a shower, finding that I am not hungry because I am not doing anything but sitting, I consider what I've done to myself. Will it be worth it in the end? Will I be transformed?

But what precisely am I transforming into? It's tempting to think that I'm becoming the person I would have been in different circumstances, but I don't know that to be true. Physically, perhaps I would have looked different, but had I never gained weight, would I have been who I am now? I don't know. I can pretend all I want that words would have called to me anyway, that I would be thoughtful and concerned about the environment, socially responsible and all of that, but I don't know that for a fact. I don't really even know who I am now, sometimes, so it's hard to say if I would have been the same.

But I guess I'm just thinking about how wondrous things can sometimes emerge from tragedy. When that happens, does it make the tragedy easier or harder to bear? For those of us whose lives are shaped by tragedy, what does that make us? Do the ghosts and memories we carry make us better than anyone else, or just different? Why is it that some of us react differently?

Here I am wandering again—I'll stop now, since I'm not getting anywhere. But I'll leave with this final thought. All our lives are touched by tragedy or darkness of some sort. How we react to that darkness reveals aspects of our true selves that we might never before have seen, for good or for ill. Out of the darkness comes illumination, and it is up to us what we do with that knowledge.

As I healed, I slowly incorporated exercise and cooking back into my life, not realizing until then how much I'd missed those activities. Returning to my routines made me happy, although once the wraps came off my arms, I found they still looked very heavy. It seemed I had set my expectations too high, as usual.

In an effort to focus on the positive, the next time I took a shower, I paid more attention to my arms. Oddly, I discovered a change in my elbow crease, although it didn't bother me. I also immediately noticed one very good thing: my arms no longer radically changed shape when I moved them. When down, no baggy folds of skin pooled around my elbows. When out to my sides, the loose skin no longer swayed independently. When over my head, the skin no longer bunched around my shoulders.

My heart lifted. Maybe it had been silly of me to be so focused on removing some of this evidence of my earlier weight. After all, what did I gain from it? Certainly no extra strength or ability. But I did have a new sense of freedom, daydreaming about wearing short sleeves or even something sleeveless, without baggy skin immediately exposing my past. Now I could choose when to reveal my history.

I agreed with Shelly: the experience was worthwhile. I went to bed with a light heart, wondering what further transformations life might bring.

22 Opening to Happiness

Winter 2007 to Fall 2008—age 30–32, 130–135 pounds

February 3, 2007

And then while out skiing, I felt an upwelling of sheer happiness and delight. It took me a bit to recognize the feeling, so unfamiliar in daily life, but it was there, an old friend ready to greet me. It came partly from the exquisite beauty of the day, for everything was winter perfect: the patches of misty blue sky, the fast-moving platinum-colored clouds carrying a few extra flurries, the purity of the landscape in its new coverlet, the trees turned into delicate fairy-like beings, the soft trilling calls of winter birds, the fat falling flakes of snow blowing onto my ready tongue and landing on my black mittens, their tiny glory revealed in stark contrast an instant before fading, melted by the residual heat of my body.

But it was more than that. It was happiness at my capability to be out in the snow, my feet plowed under at times as I forged new trails, the exertion warming but not exhausting me. Too rarely do I remember to take pleasure and joy in this newer body of mine, forgetting what it was once like. But this morning I thought of how I never would have done something like this as an adolescent because it would have been too hard to be fun. Today I found happiness in the knowledge that I not only can do these things now, but that I choose to. It was as if something clicked inside me, and I had a very clear sense of connection and recognition with Mom.

And finally, I was happy because I let myself take the time to be happy. I paused a few times to simply admire the beauty of the landscape and world around me, reveling in the morning stillness and solitude and wonder. I was reminded of Michael Pollan's description in The Omnivore's Dilemma *of how he looked at the world differently when hunting for boar or plants or fungi. For me, though, I was hunting beauty, and when you open your eyes to it, it's everywhere.*

And so I basked in my happiness, knowing it might be as ephemeral as the lives of those snowflakes on my mitten, but perhaps all the more wondrous for that. It was still with me when I came home; I did not stop skiing because I was tired of it but more because I wanted to capture some of these words bubbling within me; they, too, can easily vanish if I am not careful. Whether I have gotten the exact words I wanted I do not know; but at least I have a sense of them. And now, as I go about my day, may I feel this happiness, and be open to it, more often.

By early 2007 I had fully healed from the surgery and truly begun appreciating my body as I never had before, and not only because of my arms. My knees had also made a nearly full recovery, and although I never had returned to a natural menstrual cycle, I'd come to accept it.

The joy and delight I felt while skiing became a greater part of my life, and it helped me remember how much I had done, boosting my self-confidence and allowing me to attempt things I wouldn't have been comfortable with before.

One such adventure came in September 2008 when I traveled by myself to the Galapagos Islands. Going so far, all alone, turned out to be thrilling and nerve-wracking, as did joining a tour group where I didn't know anyone. I knew the experience would be well worth it. What I didn't expect was another insight related to weight loss.

On my first full day of the tour, we went to Bartolome Island, a barren, volcanic creation, populated only at the water's edge by a few pelicans, Sally Lightfoot crabs, a lava heron, a sea lion, and a few marine iguanas. We proceeded up the fairly steep path to the view of Pinnacle Rock. At the top, I admired the 360-degree panorama, filled with awe and also deep gratitude at being able to climb easily.

That sense heightened a few minutes later when Kate, the only other American woman in the group, joined me, breathing heavily. She carried a little extra weight but didn't seem to have any serious trouble.

We hadn't talked much, but she clearly needed to complain. "You won't believe what the guide said to me."

"What?"

"He said, 'You're a bit fat, aren't you?'"

"What?" I repeated, this time in shock, especially when I pictured our guide and his own noticeable belly.

"Yeah, I think bluntness is part of the cultural difference between us and the people here."

"I would say so." I shook my head. "That's still unbelievable, especially since he's got extra padding himself."

I debated saying something about my own weight experience, but then some of the others joined us and we resumed sightseeing. After lunch, though, as we sailed to our next island, Kate and I had the boat's deck to ourselves. With none of my own travel companions, I wanted to find ways of connecting with the others on the tour. Remembering Kate's comment from the morning, I thought sharing my experience might be a way to do that.

"Earlier, when you told me the guide's comment about you, it was kind of funny because I'd been remembering my own weight issues, and how hard that hike would have been for me a few years ago."

"What do you mean? You're not fat."

"Not now, but eight years ago I weighed 130 pounds more than I do now."

She stared at me in astonishment. "I can't imagine it. What happened? Had you been overweight for long?"

Before I knew it, I told her the whole story of my weight loss, and early childhood and adolescent experiences: how judged I felt, how hard it was to get around, the ill-fitting clothes, the shame and guilt around eating, the problems with my parents.

It had become distant enough for me to speak about matter-of-factly, but seeing her expression, it occurred to me most people had never experienced such a body or wouldn't have any idea of what being extremely overweight is truly like.

"My God, that sounds horrible!" she said when I had finished.

"It was," I admitted. Actually saying it, and having her respond sympathetically, was oddly freeing. I hadn't talked about it openly for a while, and it made me realize I had, somehow, let it go. It helped me enjoy the trip that much more.

Then in November, Jeremiah, Marie and I continued a tradition we'd developed of traveling the week of Thanksgiving, this time by going to Tucson. We stayed at a B&B owned by a woman who used to be a pastry chef and owned a French restaurant. Our hostess knew her food, and it showed.

On November 22, our first morning, we walked into the kitchen, greeted by the delicious aroma of fresh muffins and bacon. The muffins sat in a basket on the table beside some butter and jam, along with a bowl of assorted fruit and three elegant place settings, complete with cloth napkins in napkin rings.

"Good morning," we said, pleasantly dazed.

Our hostess smiled at us from where she stood at the stove tending the bacon. "Good morning. Go ahead and start, but pace yourselves because there's bacon and omelets coming."

We sat and started with the muffins, moist and warm and delicious, with bits of apple baked into them. "I'm not used to multi-course meals for breakfast," I commented as she brought over a plate of steaming, crisp bacon. "This is wonderful."

"I'm glad you think so." She left us to eat contentedly for a bit before returning with lovely golden omelets.

"Thank you so much," I said before digging in.

I savored the bites, with the eggs cooked to perfection and stuffed with cheese, peppers, scallions, and a combination of herbs. I knew I didn't need so much, but I didn't worry about it, also knowing we'd be flexible in the size and timing of other meals. Besides, I didn't want to pass up such delicious food.

Over the remaining days we had a spectacular variety of breakfasts: parfait with pumpkin granola and lots of fruit; fresh bread; ham; banana bread; puffy pancakes and pears; waffles with both maple syrup and cranberry syrup; sausage; mini quiches; savory crêpes with ham, cheese, and asparagus; and sweet crêpes loaded with apples and whipped cream. I don't think any of us had ever eaten so well for breakfast.

It made me rather introspective, as I wrote on November 26, Thanksgiving morning:

I find myself being grateful for food and my relationship to it. Now that it's been five and a half years, I can finally relax a bit on food restrictions and know that it will be okay. It's enabled me to really enjoy the breakfasts, eating them without shame for how much I'm eating or fear of gaining lots of weight. For so much of my life, if I had been presented with this sort of food, I would have only eaten tiny amounts in front of others, then felt guilty even for that while also being hungry and trying to find a way to eat more later. While I still worry a little about the impact of some of those goodies, I know it's temporary, and I'll enjoy it while I can.

That feeling allowed me to appreciate Thanksgiving more than I had in years, perhaps ever, no longer conflicted by the holiday message of indulgence, and other voices encouraging restriction. My joy, though, would soon be tempered by sorrow.

23 Weight History
Late 2008 to Fall 2009—age 34, 130–135 pounds

December 16, 2008

One of my former senior youth group advisors, Paul, died a couple of days ago, and it hit me pretty hard. Jeremiah and I had been to visit not long ago to share our thoughts about losing a parent as a young adult, since Paul's kids are now facing that. At the end of the visit, Paul also told me he really wanted me to try to get my poetry published. It's a lot to carry, and I need to give myself permission, sometimes, to acknowledge that, and just breathe and sigh, and admit to grief.

Like today, at work I was listening to Andy Happel's "On Metal Strings," and it made me think about Paul and how important music was to him. And now he'll never get to play anything again, or listen to the music of others. And even if I ever do get published, he won't be here to see it. But I do want to pursue the poetry route, since it was the last thing he asked me to do, or encouraged me to try. Yet no matter what positive aspect I take from this, it doesn't change the fact that he's gone, or that his kids no longer have a father, or his wife Noel a husband. And it doesn't change me wishing things were different.

December 21, 2008

Winter Solstice and day of Paul's memorial service
The authenticity of Paul's life really struck me during his memorial service. I haven't always been that way, I suppose because I haven't always known who I was. But only by being true to myself can I possibly hope to share that self in a true, meaningful way with another.

It started me thinking of writing a story based on my experience, about an orphaned young woman trying to find her way through the world and in order to come out safely she has to acknowledge and remember what her mother taught her and understand what parts of her were inherited from her mother.

In early 2009, per Paul's request, I submitted some poetry but didn't have any success with publication. Discouraged on that front, by June I returned to the story idea I'd had at the memorial service, but I didn't quite know how to begin. Seeking inspiration, for the first time I looked at the three-ring binders Dad had given me years before: Mom's diaries.

As I picked one at random, tears sprang to my eyes. I could picture, vividly, Mom sitting at the kitchen table, binder open in front of her, long hair framing her face, light reflecting off her glasses, expression intent as she leaned over to write a few notes about the day. After so many years, it still astonished me how quickly grief could overtake me, making me miss her terribly, wanting to reach out and touch the picture of her in my mind.

With a deep breath, I opened the binder and found another surprise. Unlike the stream-of-consciousness rambling in my journal, Mom had a very specific method for her diary, although later I discovered that entries in some of the other binders took a more free-form approach. In these early ones, though, she had divided each sheet into columns: date and weather; her morning temperature and weight; how she felt physically and emotionally; sometimes what she did for exercise; and finally a small space, maybe an inch or two, for anything noteworthy about the day.

The binder had entries from the mid-1980's, and out of curiosity, I searched for what she said about my first visit to Baxter State Park and the hike up Katahdin in 1986. I found three entries relating to the trip:

8/30 (nice day): packing for Mt. K—left by 9—arrived about 2. Walked to Abol Falls, <u>drove</u> to Roaring Brook, took Nature Trail, played Yahtzee.

8/31 (beautiful, cool, breezy, but nice): eggs/homefries/sausage for breakfast—Climbed Mt. Katahdin—Abol Trail (!) 10 hours.

9/1 (warm, 75-80): watched chipmunks, filmed, headed home, unpacked.

Amazing how such a long, difficult day had been distilled into such a brief note. I knew she had wanted to type up the diaries and use the chance to flesh them out, but she ran out of time.

Curious, I scanned more entries to see what she considered worth mentioning. I found a lot about visits with family and friends, church activities, gardening in the summer, teaching the rest of the year.

Then an entry on September 18, 1988 took me off guard: "Erica began Weight Watchers."

Again, those brief words brought back a flood of memories, this time not happy ones. How I hadn't been able to climb Katahdin that summer for the second year in a row. How my failure seemed to trigger something in my parents because not long afterwards Dad told me I *had* to go to Weight Watchers—and Mom backed him up. My humiliation at that first meeting in the basement of a nearby church, being the youngest person by far, and being weighed. Resentful for being forced to attend, I grew rebellious, but at the same time I wanted to succeed. When the Weight Watchers leaders asked about our goal for losing weight, my immediate response, then and always: to be able to climb Katahdin again.

Once past my initial reaction, I realized Mom's note shouldn't have surprised me. She clearly tracked her own weight, terrified of getting diabetes after having seen both of her grandmothers suffer from it. Knowing that, and given how much pressure she'd put on me about my weight, it made sense for her to clearly note my first attempt at losing.

Except she tracked much more, writing about every time I went to Weight Watchers, and whether I'd gained or lost weight. I found entries like:

11/21/88: "Erica to Wt. Watchers. Gained ½ lb. She was upset."

12/5/88: "Lost 2½ lbs!! She was very excited."

12/12/88: "Same weight. She wasn't surprised."

3/16/89: "Erica to Wt. Watchers. Gained 2 lbs. on break-through diet. Upset. Left. Not sure she wants to continue."

I hadn't returned to the meetings after March 1989, at least not right away. But after regaining lost weight, I made my own decision to try again, as Mom noted on June 29, 1989: "Erica back to W.W. Gained back all but 1 lb. Wants to lose again. I wish her the best."

I read it all avidly, remembering bits and pieces as I went, along with other major events, such as our dog, Alaski, being put to sleep, buying our Amiga 500 computer, Jeremiah going to camp, and more.

Wanting to share some of those memories, I asked Dad, "Did you know Mom used to write about when I went to Weight Watchers?"

"No, I didn't, or if I did, I forgot."

"She also wrote about your weight-loss competitions with Marcel."

He laughed. "Those I remember! I got pretty competitive about it."

I snorted. "That's an understatement." Dad hated losing any kind of game or competition.

"True. I don't think Marcel was very happy with me." He paused. "But as far as your weight, you know we were concerned for your health, but we also worried you might have a hard time getting a job."

"Really?" This possibility had never occurred to me.

"Oh, yeah, especially once you entered high school. Clearly it wasn't a problem, and we shouldn't have put our concern on you, but I don't think we knew what to do. Neither of us had been heavy when we were young, and we felt like we were failing you as parents somehow."

His revelation tipped me off-balance. All these years, I had focused so much on my reactions to being heavy, on my pain and anger. I hadn't once considered what the experience of raising a fat daughter might have been like for my parents.

"I had no idea," I said. "I wish Mom were here to talk to about it."

"Me, too."

That feeling only intensified when I later saw my chiropractor, Dr. Lindsey. Since she had become quite close to the family, especially Mom, I mentioned my project of going through Mom's diaries and finding notes about my weight.

"Do you want to know what I remember?" Dr. Lindsey asked.

"Um, okay." I didn't know what to expect.

"Your mom used to come in here, all upset about your weight and how much you were gaining, and I'd try to talk her down, to remind her you were a smart girl and you'd lose weight when you were ready."

I held silent a moment, stunned. "I had no idea. Thank you for talkng to her."

"Well, I imagined how it must have been for you, with her constantly picking at it, like Chinese water torture."

"Yeah, that's about how it felt sometimes."

The insights fueled my desire to go through the diaries, but now with a new focus: to piece together my weight history and journey and write it out, to puzzle out for myself why and when everything had happened.

I found more and more. How Mom got me sugar-free candy but bought regular candy for Jeremiah. How she gave me books as a reward for exercise, arranged for me to see a counselor, came with me to Shapedown, had me try a yeast-free diet, and more. Some of it I'd forgotten, or forgotten when it happened. I began to understand how it all played out, tracing the roots of my insecurities in her own fears.

Next I found this note, from August 5, 1992, the eventful day when Mom found me with candy I'd bought in secret, which then led to our conversation about weight issues in general:

> Erica and I had a long talk about her seeing counselors for her weight. She isn't happy about any of this. I have decided to drop everything for a good long while.

I browsed her diaries through 1994, the year of my high school graduation, but didn't find much else. Next I turned to my own journals. While losing weight, I had typed up the journals from 1991 to 2001, an enormous effort but something I now appreciated. Having it on the computer meant I could easily skim and do word searches on things like "weight", "diet", "food", and "exercise." It proved enlightening.

June 25, 2009

I've now read journal entries over a ten-year period that all mention weight, and it's astonishing to see the difference in my attitude after Mom's death. It's obvious that I changed, since that's when I actually lost weight, but I'd never read the condensed version like that. It also made me realize how much my relationship with Dad has improved, I think because we've both changed. I'd forgotten how hurt I was by some of what he said, or didn't say, and I'm so very glad we've gotten past that. I am grateful for what we have now.

August 2, 2009

I've gotten back to working on "A Losing Battle", and I'm still thoroughly engaged in it. It feels a little odd to say I'm enjoying writing about all my struggles, but in a way I am because I know the ending is a good one. More than that, I'm absorbed when I work on it, losing track of time and able to put aside other concerns, at least for a while.

What's also rather interesting is trying to make some cohesive shape out of it all, to understand how things connected and make it flow reasonably well. It's more difficult than it would seem because while the patterns may be there, I need to look from a higher point to see them. But it's well worth the effort.

Going through my hand-written journals took longer, but I kept at it, fascinated to rediscover weight and food issues but also other life events I'd lost track of. I didn't consider doing anything with the information, though, until I visited my friend Clara.

"Have you thought about trying to publish your book?" she asked.

I mulled over my answer as I watched her kids run around. "No I hadn't. I'm mostly writing it for myself, or maybe anyone else in the family who's interested."

"You should think about publishing, since it's such an inspirational story, and it might really help other kids, more than just ones who are overweight."

The idea had a certain appeal. "I'll think about it."

"Maybe you could start by keeping a blog about what you're thinking of for food, and about your weight issues these days. It will help build up a following and get you used to having other people read your work."

"Good idea. Thanks."

As I wrote about my losing process, I realized Clara had a point—it did feel inspirational. I started seriously considering the idea of eventual publication, which prompted me to start a blog in late October.

It all seemed to be going well, until the end of December when events at work threw me for a loop.

24 Finding My Path

December 2009 to Summer 2011—age 33–35, 125–135 pounds

December 23, 2009

It's been a trying day. This morning I got up feeling not that great (sneezy, sore throat), and I woke late, just in time to go to work. Then it ended not so well with my review with my manager. At an earlier review he said my documents were considered the standard of excellence in the department, but now we have a new process. Per the new review criteria, I now meet expectations, and that's it. That was largely what I expected, but I still wasn't excited about it. But then we talked about the upcoming year, and he wants me to focus on fewer products so I can be a really good Product Manager instead of a "mediocre" one. That phrase really bothered me.

The review comments encouraged me to do some self-evaluation during my holiday vacation. After over ten years, I thought I had achieved more than "mediocre" at my job, but I also realized my heart wasn't quite in it. Much as I still enjoyed many aspects of my work, I'd started traveling more, something I'd never wanted to do except for fun. I had always been a homebody, and I found it increasingly stressful to be away more often.

Traveling for work also made it harder for me to participate in activities outside of my job. I had to miss some worship service planning meetings at church. Finding time to visit friends and family became challenging. I worried about leaving my cats alone so much, and I also had less time to write.

Then, when Shelly and I met for lunch not long after Christmas, she reminded me of another casualty of the work situation by asking, "Anything new on the guy front?"

I sighed and shook my head. "I don't even feel like I have the energy for dating, and when I occasionally do, it can be really hard scheduling times to get together since I'm not around a lot, and the travel can sometimes be last-minute."

"It sounds like work is stressing you out. Do you think you'll look for something else?"

I'd been giving the possibility a lot of thought. "Maybe, but the thing is, I'm not sure I want to do this type of work at all. Even when Mom died ten years ago I kept worrying about that." I paused, giving the tightness in my throat a chance to relax. "She always knew she wanted to be a teacher, and she did work she loved. But I've never been passionate about being in the computer field. It just happened. If I only have another fifteen years, like she did, I don't know if I want to be doing something I don't really love."

Shelly's eyes looked suspiciously bright as she asked, "So what do you want to do?"

I laughed. "That's the million dollar question. In a dream world, I'd love to be able to support myself with writing, but I know it's not going to happen. I want to do something that directly helps people, but I don't have any more specifics. So I've made an appointment with a career counselor, and hopefully she can help me figure it out."

Over the next few days before the meeting with the counselor, I looked at local colleges and community colleges, to get a sense of available options. Unfortunately, my confusion only increased as I realized how many courses I found interesting.

"Like what?" the counselor asked when I explained my dilemma.

"Let's see. I've thought about being a minister, grief counselor, dietitian, radiologist, marine biologist, environmental scientist, and maybe more I'm forgetting."

"That's actually good—some people don't have any idea, or they only like one idea, which can be limiting. But we'll do some exercises to help identify not only what you want to do but what type of work might suit you. So the first thing is to come back next time with a list of six accomplishments you're most proud of, and a paragraph about each one."

When I sat down to make the list, my weight loss immediately sprang to mind. Working on the book had allowed me to finally recognize pride in that accomplishment, and how it became a turning point in my life. More than the difference in pounds, my whole outlook had changed. I realized how much I could do, and that instead of being a bit player, I could be in charge of my own life.

I shared those thoughts with the counselor, and as we continued the process, I realized I wanted to find work that would dovetail with the book and help others develop a healthier relationship to food and themselves. All the introspection, though, brought up some difficult questions for me.

My impetus to lose weight, and eventually discover what work I might truly love, had all been triggered by Mom's death. Had she lived, would I have ever lost weight? If I hadn't, where would I be in life? Would I have realized my weight didn't define me, and I deserved love no matter how many pounds registered on the scale? What did it say about me that I could find happiness out of so much pain and anguish?

The thoughts plagued me for a time until I spoke with someone at church about it. He said, "But that's how it's supposed to work. Out of death comes life and new growth."

I hadn't thought of it that way before, and it helped. "You're right."

I had not, after all, been responsible for Mom's death, nor could I change it. I could only control my reaction to such events, and I decided I wanted my response to be exactly this: finding meaning and joy in my life, for as long as I might have it.

Those thoughts allowed me to let go of the guilt and sorrow and plunge into possibilities with excitement, although it did mean putting writing on the back seat for a while.

"So I'm thinking of being a dietitian and starting with the dietetic technician program at Southern Maine Community College," I told my friend Clara on a visit after church one day.

"That sounds like a great idea," she said. "And community college is definitely the way to go - it's so much less expensive."

"The ironic part is how much I hated the idea of talking to anyone about my weight when I was younger, and yet here I am now wanting to be in the business of working with people on food and weight issues."

She gave me a big smile. "I'm so proud of you for doing what you're passionate about. Besides, your experience makes you the perfect person for this."

"Thanks. I don't know if I'm being brave or stupid, but it feels nice to think about doing something that will actually help people." I paused, folding my legs under me on the couch. "It's so strange, though, to think about going into business for myself. I never thought I'd have the self-confidence for it, but when I told the career counselor about my ideas, she said I'm thinking like an entrepreneur."

"That's so awesome. And you'll be great at it."

"I hope so. Now I need to talk to some dietitians to find out what's involved."

Once I did that, though, all my excitement drained away. "I don't know what to do," I told the career counselor, despondent. "In order for me to become a dietitian, I'd need a whole new Bachelor's degree, plus a year internship. The internships are pretty scarce, and I'd have to pay for it, too. Then after all that, my best bet of getting a job would be at a hospital, nursing home, or correctional facility, mostly writing meal plans per FDA regulations. Which is exactly what I *don't* want to do."

"So that's why you're exploring your options. Didn't you say you have more calls lined up, with other people in the health field?"

"Yes." I felt a little down, wanting to wallow in misery.

But finally I motivated myself enough to talk to someone else. She mentioned the name of a weight loss coach. I cheered up. It sounded much more like what I might want. Then in talking to the coach, I learned about something even more promising.

"It's called the Am I Hungry?® Mindful Eating program," I told Shelly, excited all over again. "It's all about mindful eating, to help people figure out why they're eating, and really pay attention to when they're hungry instead of wanting to eat for some other reason, like they're bored or stressed. It's definitely not a diet, but a group program with some structure and guidance."

"That does sound like a good fit."

"And even better, a lot of materials have already been developed by Dr. Michelle May, the woman who created the program. So it's basically a license, where she trains other people to be facilitators, and then I lead the program here, since she's in Arizona. Now I want to read her book and make sure it's what I think it is, but I feel like this is a much better direction than being a dietitian."

My excitement grew when I read Dr. May's book, *Eat What You Love, Love What You Eat.* I could relate to so much of it, since it echoed my own approach of paying attention to what my body told me over what someone else told me to do.

Shortly afterwards I prepared for my annual trip to Baxter State Park, my twenty-fifth summer in a row. To commemorate it, I put together a small album of photos from all those years, and seeing the visual record of changes in myself motivated me even more.

While at Baxter, Jeremiah and I decided to hike Doubletop, not feeling quite up for Katahdin. I had to stop a lot to catch my breath, not having prepared for hiking, but I made it. When we reached the second of the double peaks, I took a long moment to savor the view and my ability to see it, which I still found astonishing. As I later reflected in my journal:

Because it really is amazing what I did. I can recognize that more clearly now, and finally acknowledge what effort and will it all took. And I can now, looking back, seek to recapture that feeling, at least from time to time, and also revel in knowing that it has become so much of my expectation that I don't think about what I do on a daily basis. There is wonder in that, too. Never, ever as an adolescent would I have guessed that one day I wouldn't think twice about exercising every day, or wearing a short-sleeved shirt, or walking up a flight of stairs with a heavy backpack, or carrying heavy bags from the Farmers' Market because fresh produce would prove as irresistible as candy once was.

Not that everything is as I imagined. I've come to acknowledge certain truths: I will never be naturally athletic; my legs will never look the way I once hoped they would; I will carry my scars and stretch marks to the grave; I will never know what it's like to have smooth, taut skin in certain areas.

But I'm okay with that because in the end, the reality is far richer than I ever would have guessed. These days I don't constantly think about the limitations of my body. It isn't a source of unending shame, frustration, or embarrassment. I know I'm not model-thin, but I'm okay with that. My body does what I need it to, and for that I give great thanks. While I may not take or have as much time anymore for reflection, it is still something essential to me, as these pages show. I will try to be better about remembering in general where I have come from, to thus appreciate all the more the distance traveled and gain strength from it, to know I can meet whatever challenges lie ahead.

I have two legs that can take me where I need to go. My feet are small but work fine and are even, in some lights, cute. My arms are strong enough to carry bags of groceries, cradle a baby, or give someone a long hug. My hands, always my pride and joy, are capable of so much, allowing me to create in so many ways. My ears hear all that I need and want, including the voices of loved ones and music that stirs my soul. My stomach may not be flat but it is strong, and if I listen to it, it tells me all I need to know about hunger. My mouth expresses so much, with a smile or words or melodies, and I can safely eat all manner and textures of foods. My eyes, a marvel of evolution, take in the wonders of everything around me. My skin, wrinkled as it is, is capable of feeling so much, sometimes pain but also exquisite pleasure.

I once tried to shun the physical world, live only in my head, but no longer. My body ties me to this world, its atoms composed of stardust and the molecules of my ancestors, and this is all to be celebrated, not ignored. I thank this body for providing me with so much, and I only hope I have many more years in which to appreciate it.

When I returned from Baxter, I signed up for the Am I Hungry?® (AIH) Mindful Eating facilitator training. I immediately knew I had found the right approach, not only because I agreed with the principles, but because the training included a lot of useful business information I needed.

Before starting, though, I wondered how much benefit I would get from another part of the training process: going through the program myself. After all, how much could I have to learn after figuring out so much on my own?

The smugness quickly got knocked out of me. Dr. May and the other facilitators had their own insights to share, ideas and approaches I'd never considered. The experience also showed me how restrictive some of my habits had become. Yet it only served to excite me more, thinking I'd be able to learn as well as teach. I couldn't wait to hold my own AIH session.

Given the holidays and my travel schedule, though, that had to wait until the spring of 2011. Excited but nervous, I held the first workshop on April 20, with seven people signed up. What if it went badly? As soon as I started, though, any concerns disappeared. Knowing a couple of the women helped, as did the fact that the others mostly appeared to be open to what I said, and everyone appreciated knowing that they weren't alone with their problems.

I proceeded with more confidence, sharing my own experience when it made sense, letting the participants know I could understand some of the challenges they faced. Leading the class also helped me realize I still had my own issues to work on, especially concerning body image, and I could use some of the AIH strategies to help with it.

The best part, though, came when I read the feedback forms.

One read: "I really enjoyed the workshop. Erica's personal stories made a big difference in our motivation to keep on going. I am very impressed with the book, and was able to use the workshop to ask questions, clarify, and listen to others' experience…. I love the philosophy of the program, and really feel like it is something I can continue on forever."

Another commented: "I loved this workshop mostly for being so practical, no-nonsense and—most of all—nonjudgmental. Every other diet approach I had tried before involved some degree of judgment and many rules—and some type of 'complications' of counting, measuring, weighing, checking off—allowed or forbidden foods. I knew I needed to re-learn to trust my own body to know what it needs, wants, when and how much. I was skeptical if such a seemingly oversimplified approach could work for a lifelong chocoholic like me—and discovered to my amazement that it did. In fact, it's the first eating approach that has broken my chocolate addiction without putting chocolate in the 'bad food' category. I feel so well-nourished now, that I rarely want it anymore—and if I do, I can enjoy it and then stop! Thank you!"

Knowing how much it helped them, and having heard other comments during the workshops about being able to let go of feelings of shame and guilt around food, made me incredibly happy. I couldn't wait to do more.

Only one major concern dampened my excitement: my present job. With the unpredictable nature of the travel, and the frequency, I knew I couldn't reliably hold an eight-week AIH session, not if I didn't even know when I'd be home. But now that I had discovered what I wanted to do, I wouldn't let it go.

At the same time, I couldn't simply quit my job because the AIH work would only be part-time, especially at the start, and not enough to pay bills. I decided to supplement AIH by becoming a certified health coach through the Institute for Integrative Nutrition®, and I signed up for the dietetic technician program at SMCC. I hoped that, if necessary, between school loans and other part-time efforts I'd be able to make ends meet.

Then, with my heart in my throat, I told my manager at the end of May, "I'm not willing to travel. If you tell me it's a requirement for my job, I'll have to resign."

At first he didn't know what to say. "Are you sure?"

Not really, I thought, but out loud I said, "Yes, I'm sure."

"All right. I'll see what I can do."

I hadn't known what to expect, but when the HR person in my office suggested the idea of working part-time, I grew excited. If I could still do some work there, but without the constant travel, and have some extra time for the mindful eating work and book, that would be ideal.

After multiple discussions, my manager and I settled on a proposal. I'd work thirty hours a week, enough to keep benefits, Tuesday through Friday, with no travel except a single yearly conference. My last hurdle: discussing the proposal with our CEO to see if he would support it.

On July 6, I had a phone conversation with the CEO. After explaining the situation, and how I wanted to change my role so I could also do other activities where I could directly help people, he said, "I can appreciate that. I also appreciate that you've been here for almost twelve years, and your experience is truly invaluable. We can iron out details later, but I'd say you can assume we'll work it out."

Elated, I felt confident enough to relax and cancel my enrollment at SMCC. Brimming with excitement, I headed to Baxter State Park on July 9.

Epilogue

July 10, 2011—age 35, 125 pounds

At Baxter, Jeremiah, Marie, and I planned to hike a big loop, about nine miles in total: Chimney Pond trail to North Basin cut over to Blueberry Knoll, then back to North Basin trail, Hamlin Ridge, and Chimney Pond before returning to the Roaring Brook campsite.

We had good weather, sunny with a few clouds that quickly cleared up. On the first part of the trail, we made very good time, and I felt fine. I had prepared more than the year before, and it paid off. But when we arrived at Blueberry Knoll, Jeremiah sat down somewhat heavily.

"Are you okay?" I asked. He didn't seem his usual energetic self.

"I don't know. I'm really tired for some reason."

"Are you drinking enough?"

"I think so, and I got a reasonable amount of sleep." He shrugged. "I'll be okay."

We headed off to Hamlin Ridge, a much more challenging trail. Not quite as bad as Cathedral, but steep enough, and as we rapidly passed the tree line and came out of the forest cover, we enjoyed amazing views. But neither Jeremiah nor Marie wanted to do much of the trail.

For the first time in memory, I found myself able and wanting to do more than them. I even thought I could do the whole mountain, although I knew I didn't want to attempt it on my own. But I could do a little more.

Without thinking about it I asked, "Do you mind if I go on for a bit while you wait here?"

"Knock yourself out."

As I headed up, often using my hands as well as feet to get over the rocks, I marveled. Here I was, choosing to go higher, without care or concern for what it would be like coming back down, simply trusting I could do it. It felt incredibly liberating. As I climbed higher and saw more and more spectacular views, I couldn't stop smiling, simply delighted with the whole experience.

Eventually I stopped, not wanting to make Jeremiah and Marie wait too long. But I paused for a moment to appreciate the sights and reflect.

I remembered, then, how Dad had once told me, "There was a time when you were fearless."

He had been referring to my early childhood, maybe four or five years old, a time when I would do anything. Up to then I'd never had cause to feel afraid, but more, something in my personality seemed geared that way. If I wanted to do something, nothing would keep me from it.

After I gained weight, though, my fearlessness vanished. I had wondered, did it simply get crushed beneath the layers of fat, spark extinguished beyond any hope of resurrection? Or might it emerge, phoenix-like, granting me the freedom to soar above everything?

I'd come close to recovering that feeling before, once when I climbed Katahdin to scatter Mom's ashes, and a couple of other instances, but it had never been quite the same—until now. I hadn't been looking for it, but perhaps that's why I found it. Like I was four years old again, unscarred by the world, ready for anything, not just on the trail but on my new life's path.

Fearless.

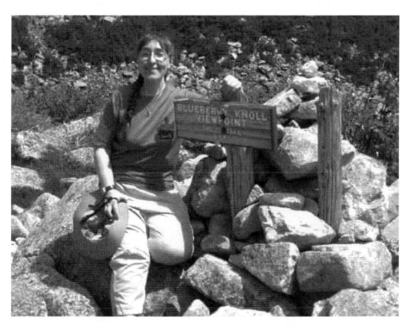

Erica at Blueberry Knoll, July 2011

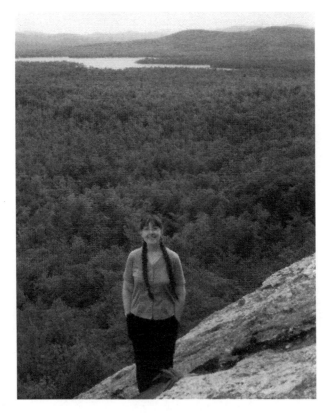

Erica on Bald Pate Mountain, summer 2011

Acknowledgments

I owe many thanks to all my family and friends who appear in the book, but I'd especially like to thank my parents, my brother, and Shelly.

I also want to acknowledge others who didn't quite make it into the book. In no particular order:

My friends Allison, Matt, and Doe, who offered support and editing during the writing process.

The Portland Writer's Meetup group, for all the very useful feedback, particularly those who read outside of the group, and especially Roger Pepper, who read and helped with the whole publication process.

Kitty Werner, who came up with such a wonderful cover and overall design.

Members of my church, Allen Avenue Unitarian Universalist, for giving me a safe place to share some of my experience and helping me cultivate my enjoyment of lay-led worship. Especially thanks to members of my spiritual enrichment group for general support and friendship, members of the Worship Committee, and those on the Caring Connection and others who assisted during my recuperation from cosmetic surgery.

Teachers who encouraged my love of writing, particularly: Barbara Moore, Kathy Bartley, and Jake Laferriere.

Dr. Michelle May, for creating the Am I Hungry?® Mindful Eating program and allowing me to be part of it.

Joshua Rosenthal and Lindsey Smith and others at the Institute for Integrative Nutrition® for providing such a wonderful health coaching program and book course.

Too numerous to name, all the authors who have inspired me and given me much delight in reading.

And last but definitely not least, Gov. Percival Baxter, for creating Baxter State Park for the state of Maine, and to all of those who have helped preserve his vision and keep the park and Katahdin a place of unchanging beauty.

About the Author Erica L. Bartlett

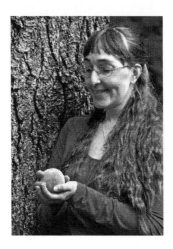

Erica L. Bartlett is, among other things, an author, certified health coach, and licensed facilitator for the Am I Hungry?® Mindful Eating program. She has been published in magazines, keeps a weekly blog about weight and food issues, and has had blog posts published on www.AmIHungry.com. When she's not writing, she enjoys many other activities, including reading, cooking, baking, walking, hiking, traveling, watching movies, listening to music, volunteering, and visiting with family and friends. She lives in Portland, Maine, with her two cats.

Printed in Great Britain
by Amazon